GET YOUR FREE BONUS NOW!

20 MINUTES HOME TRAINING

Strength Training Over 40
Step-to-Step Guide to Get Fit and Move Pain Free

Alessandro Villanucci

RESISTANCE MACHINE

Push Exercises   **25**

Chest Press   26
Shoulder Press   30
Pec Fly   33
Chest Flyers at Cable Machine   36

Pull Exercises   **41**

Seated Row   41
Lat Pulldown   44

Core Exercises   **47**

Abdominals Machine   46

Arms Exercises   **49**

Cable Bicep Curl   49
Cable Tricep Push down   52

Leg Exercises   **54**

Leg Press   54
Lying Leg Curl   57
Seated Leg Curl   62
Leg Extension   65

FREE WEIGHTS

Push Exercise   69

DB Chest Press   68
DB Flys   72
DB Overhead Press   74
DB Arnold Press   77

Pull Exercises   80

DB Row   83
BB Row   82
DB Pullover   87

Core Exercises   90

Plank Dumbbell   90
Drag Renegade Row   93

Arms Exercises   95

Bicep Curl   95
DB Skullcrusher   98

Leg Exercises   103

BB Squat   103
BB Hip Thrust   107
BB RDL   110
DB Lunge   113

BODYWEIGHT

Push Exercises — 118

Push-ups — 118
Dips — 121
Pike push-ups — 124

Pull Exercises — 126

Chin-ups — 126
Inverted Rows — 129

Core Exercises — 131

Plank — 131
Side Plank — 134

Leg Exercises — 136

Box Pistol Squat — 136
Bulgarian Split Squat — 138
Glute Bridge Stability — 140
Ball Leg Curl — 143

BULLETPROOFING EXERCISES

Ankle	**146**
Tibialis Raise	146
Calf Raise	148
Knee	**150**
Patrick Step-up	150
Reverse Nordic Curl	153
Nordic Curl	159
ATG Split Squat	162
Hips	**165**
Knee raises	165
BB RDL	168
Shoulders	**172**
DB External Rotation	173
Band Pull Apart	175

Copyright© 2022 By Alessandro Villanucci All Rights Reserved

This book is copyright protected. It ix only for personal use. You cannot amend, distribute, sell, use, quote or paraphrase any part of the content within this book, without the consent of the author or publisher.

Under no circumstances will any blame or legal responsibility be held against the publisher, or author, for any damages, reparation, or monetary loss due to the information contained within this book, either directly or indirectly

Disclaimer Notice:

Please note the entertainment purposes only. Al effort has been executed to present accurate, up to date, reliable,complete information No warranties of any kind are declared or implied. Readers acknowledge hat the author is not engaged in the rendering of legal, financial, medical or professional advice The content within this book has been derived from various sources. Please consult licensed professional before attempting any techniques outlined in this book, By reading this document, the reader agrees that under no circumstance is the responsible for any losses, direct or indirect, that are incurred as a result of the use of the information contained within this document, including, but not limited to, error, comissions, or inaccuracies.

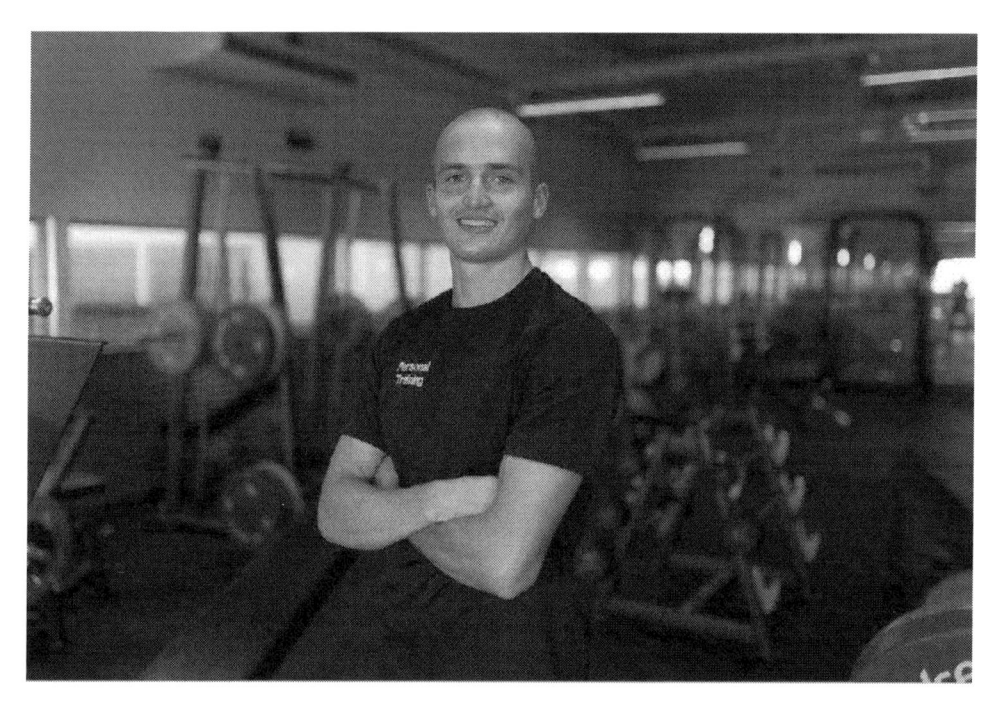

Hi, my name is Alessandro, and I wrote this guide to help you to train independently and to perform exercises correctly.

WHY READING THIS BOOK?

Would you get your physique as good as it was in your 20s?

Sick of being tired after a ramp of stairs?

Would you start going to the gym but are not sure where to start?

Would you get rid of your belly without wasting time doing useless exercises?

Simply put, this book will be your Personal Trainer in the gym. This will be your guide to help you create your own workout by giving you core principles of how to structure the training based on your goals, and a guide on how to perform exercises correctly.

Nowadays, there is a lot of information about exercises and gym workouts. Probably too much. It can be overwhelming and misleading at times. In fact, it makes fitness more complicated than it needs to be. This book aims to make your way into fitness and gym workouts easy and effective. Training for general health, muscle gain and fat loss is very simple.

This book will teach you:

- **How to Plan a Workout in the Gym**
- **The 7 Key Rules of Training**
- **The 3 Questions You Should Ask Yourself to Plan your Fitness Journey**
- **50+ Exercises with Images and Teaching Points**
- **10 Bulletproofing exercises to live and move Pain free**
- **BONUS: 5 Healthy lifestyle Hacks to 10x your Health**

This book is for you if:

- You are a beginner that just started the fitness journey.
- You have been going to the gym for a while and you want to step up your training with guidance and plenty of tips all in one single book.
- You are looking for a full guide on how to perform bodyweight, free weight and resistance machine in a safe and effective way but do not know where to start?

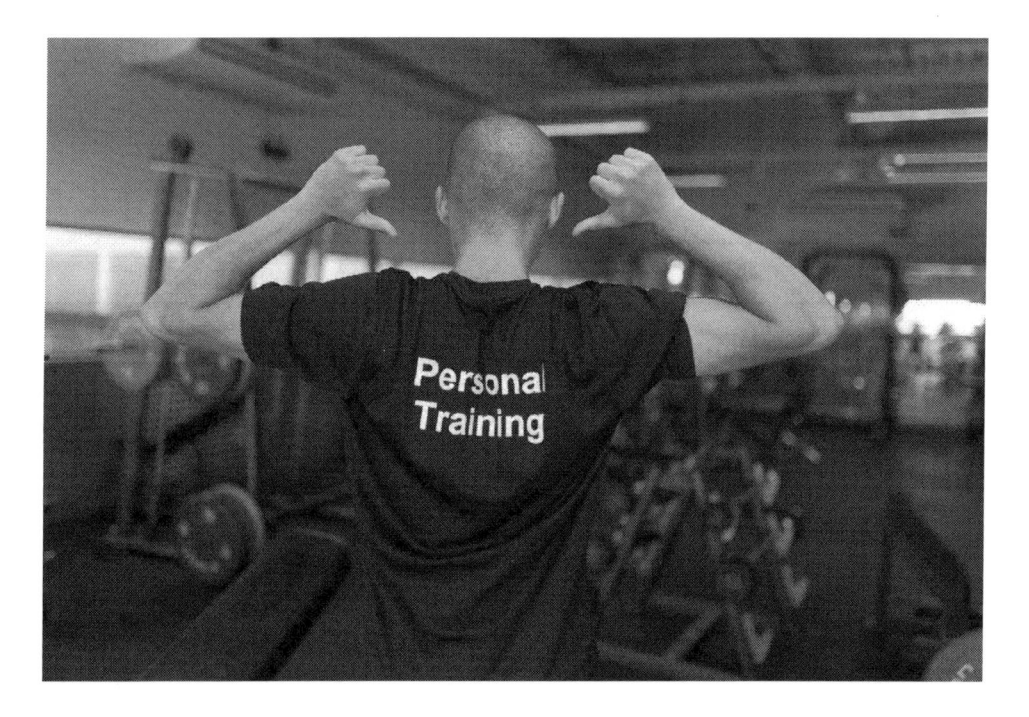

Looking at books about fitness and exercise, I noticed a gap in the market. Most of the fitness books are divided in three categories:

- Some of them are very basic that do not provide great value when it comes to perform an exercise. These books are of great help to get an idea of the benefits of exercise but often they only show a dozens of exercises without explaining how many sets and reps, how many times a week, how to progress them….

- Some of them are too advanced and not easily comprehensible unless you are a gym enthusiast. In fact, these books are (personally) amazing for personal trainers or people addicted to.

- Last one is the category that promote quick and easy 5 min routine to get shredded in 12 weeks. Unfortunately, these types of books do not provide great value. In fact, they often create illusions and false expectations to new gym-goers.

- Moreover, not many books talk about training over 40. When they do, they do not consider the challenges you might face. Your body is likely not strong, healthy, and young like when you were in your 20. Moreover, you might have some work-life balance problem to manage, low energy level, some injuries during the years and lower level of mobility.

- This book will show you the exercises that are good for you, and how to do them effectively

BENEFITS OF STRENGTH TRAINING OVER 40

Regardless of your fitness goals, (Losing weight, health reasons, gain muscle etc. etc.) these are 10 reasons why strength training must be a priority.

1. It creates stronger muscles. As you might imagine, lifting weight will make you stronger overtime. The ability of staying consistent and executing the exercises with proper technique will be effective to create stronger muscle. Having stronger muscle means you can move pain free, live better and enjoy all the activities that make your life worth living. Moreover, you will also get aesthetic movement reducing body fat and building more lean mass. Ribeiro and colleagues (2022) found that it will also increase cardiorespiratory system, especially in overweight people.

2. Optimise athletic performance. As you might know, in all sports athletes spend some time in the gym to prevent injury, get stronger, faster, and more explosive. You do not have necessarily train like them. For example, you might want to start exercise to avoid being out of breath after doing stairs, to play with your kids/grandkids without having low back pain. Having more energy through the day etc. etc.

3. Optimise athletic performance. As you might know, in all sports athletes spend some time in the gym to prevent injury, get stronger, faster, and more explosive. You do not have necessarily train like them. For example, you might want to start exercise to avoid being out of breath after doing stairs, to play with your kids/grandkids without having low back pain. Having more energy through the day etc. etc.

4. Better mood and mental health. O'Connor and colleagues (2010) studied how training on a regular basis decrease the risk of anxiety among healthy individuals. It also reduces the symptoms of depression among patients with diagnosed depression.

5. More confidence. Training will make you feel better as it will improve your look and will-power overtime. In fact, O'Connor (2010) noticed improvements in self-esteem among people that started working out.

6. Decreased likelihood of health-related diseases. Cauza and colleagues (2005) analysed how strength-training (with as little of 6 sets per muscle group weekly) play an important role in preventing osteoporosis and diabetes

*4. **Improve your sleep quality.*** Working out, especially in the morning or at least 3 hours before bedtime showed significant results in sleep quality (Kuo et al. 2017). Moreover, Kuo and colleagues (2017) studied how just after 5 weeks of training some patients decreased their likelihood of sleep apnea. Richards and colleagues (2011) found that strength training, high-intensity training and walking improved total nocturnal sleep time among elderly just after 4 weeks.

*5. **Healthy ageing.*** Training, especially strength training improves cognitive function in older adults (O'Connor et al.2010)

*6. **Boosts brain function.*** Especially in older adults' exercise, both aerobic and strength training is strongly related to brain function and ability to memorise and learn new information. (Huang, Fang, Li and Chen, 2016)

*7. **Live longer.*** A stronger body is a healthier body. A healthier body live longer and age better.

ABOUT THE BOOK

This book is divided into two parts:

- The first part will teach how to plan a session, deciding what exercises, sets, reps to do and why.
- The second part is to know how to perform exercises by giving you a step-to-step guide with illustrations.

"Note: are you a woman over 40 intimidated? Read this"

By training hundreds of people and spent hours on the gym floor and studying a lot of the scientific research, I can guarantee you that:

-Maintain muscle mass long-term.

-Make your joints stronger, with less likelihood of injury and other health related problems

-Fitter as it can be considered a low-impact cardio exercise.

-Support weight loss and weight management in a sustainable way.

-Improve cardiovascular health, especially if you perform movement that

-engage many muscles at the same time.

-Help you to live longer.

Convinced? I hope so!

FIRST PART

These are the key rules you have to know before working out. Applying these rules will give you results, make training sustainable and enjoyable.

KEY RULE #1

To improve your body and fitness progressive overload and consistency are key. That means train multiple times a week and always trying to lift more, do more reps/sets and improve your technique on a regular basis.

KEY RULE #2

You should do roughly 10 sets per muscle group every week.

Bigger muscles, such as chest, quads and back might need fewer sets, while smaller muscles (biceps and triceps for example) can do a bit more

Note: as you will see when showing the exercises, most of them works many muscles at the same time. For example, squat will work your glutes and quads at the same time (and other muscle to a lesser extent), while push-ups will work your chest, triceps, and shoulder (and core to a lesser extent).It means that as a beginner, if you are looking for general fitness and nothing specific, doing 10 sets of squats and 10 sets of pushups is more than enough to have toned and strong quads, glutes and chest, triceps, and shoulders.

Obviously, if you really want to optimize your fitness and strength level you would incorporate other exercises.

KEY RULE #1

Do not move up in weight until you OWN it.

Yes, you must strive for increasing load overtime if your technique is spot on!

That means controlling the weight in all phases of the exercise, instead of mindlessly doing reps rushed and uncontrolled to finish them.

For example, it's been a few months that I have been incorporating weighted pull-ups in my training routine. They certainly look cool, and I think the technique was good too.
However, I do feel that when I do them bodyweight, I get a better back contraction on top, and I can get my chest touching the bar rather than just having my chin over the bar. Solution? As my intention when doing pull- ups is to have a stronger and bigger back, it makes more sense to drop the weight and do them bodyweight (for now) as I feel a better muscle contraction.
Bottom line: do not let your ego get in the way when performing an exercise.

KEY RULE #1

Stick with 2-3 exercises for each part (pushing exercise, pulling exercise and legs) for 4-6 weeks. Your goal is to get better at this. Stop changing your routine every week if you want to see progress.

There is nothing wrong with trying new machine in the gym. And overtime if you only do the same exercises with the same sets and reps you might be stagnate in your results. However, if you keep changing the exercises you do on a weekly basis you do not really know where

Killing yourself in the gym 6x/week while sleeping 4 hours a night and eating junk food because you "deserved it" it is not going to get you results. **When you are over 40, I would not spend endless hours in the gym.** Having a solid 3x/week training routine while sleeping 7/8 hours a night and eating non-processed foods, drinking lots of water and prioritizing proteins, vegetables and fruit will transform your body (and your well-being) within months!

KEY RULE #1

Apply the rules below from now on, even when you do not feel like it.

if you bought this book, I assumed you have some interest in getting fitter. Therefore, I think that 3 times a week for 60 minutes is an achievable target.

2- What is my goal? Athletic performance, Getting Rid of injury/Moving Pain-Free, Gain Muscle and lose weight….

Being aware of your goal is crucial, so you know how to plan your workout. For example, if you want to increase your strength you might

want to select exercises that work many muscles at the same time, doing lots of sets, performing low reps and having long test time in between. For example, doing 5 sets of 5 reps of Barbell Squat (page 102) with 3 minutes rest in between sets.

On the other hand, if you go to the gym to get rid of knee pain, you might start doing gentle exercises such as Patrick Step-up (page 149) and doing few sets of high reps (2 /3 sets of 20+ reps) to give blood flow to the area and start the healing process.

3- What is my starting point?

It varies from person to person, but you will to some extent fit into at least one of these categories:

- I" have no experience with the gym and training. Literally starting from zero."

- "I am going to do the gym (or do some sort of exercise), but not sure if I am going in the right direction."

- "I have been going consistently to the gym/doing some exercise, but I want to step up my strength and fitness."

4- Do I have any injuries/limitations?

Being aware of your physical condition, or letting your Personal Trainer know your limitations is very important.

In fact, you should never work through pain, and always find exercises and regressions that you can perform without discomfort (well,

exercising will be challenging at times, but it should not be painful for your joints when doing any exercise in the gym)

TRAINING PLAN FOR BEGINNERS

Each workout should consist of:

-Warm up (5 to 10 minutes)

-Strength session (15 to 35 minutes)

-Cardio activity (5 to 20 minutes)

-Cool Down + Stretching (5 to 10 minutes)

Warm up

-It is useful to increase the temperature of your body, so you feel warm and ready once you start training.

-It decreases the likelihood on injuries during the training.

-It is divided into two parts:

-a few minutes of cardio activity, such as incline walking, cross trainer, cycling, stair master or rowing machine.

-a few dynamic stretches or bodyweight exercises for low reps or performing the first exercise of your session with minimal load to get the

blood flow going, prepare your connective tissue and familiarize with the technique.

-DO NOT MAKE IT TOO SHORT! Do something before getting into your session. You cannot go from sitting in your office to do bench press (or whatever exercise you are planning to do) …It might lead to injury and decrease in performance as your body is not "ready" for it

-DO NOT MAKE IT TOO LONG! That is a common mistake that people do. A few minutes of cardio to get warm and one/two dynamic exercises are more than enough for 99% of people. IT should warm you up, not tire you out.
-Cardiovascular health

Strength Session

As suggested before, for beginners (and even intermediate would work) I would suggest you do 3 times a week full body because:

- You will work each muscle three times a week. That is more than enough to get results. It also means that you do not have to push so hard in every session (that is what most people think about the gym; going crazy hard every session otherwise you do not get result…that is further from the truth)

-You will have 4 rest days. Rest days from weight training does not mean rest days from activities. You can play your favorite sports, go for a walk, or even go to the gym to walk for 30 minutes at slow pace if that's what you like…

Rest days are crucial to recover from the effort done during the workout, let the muscle recover with good diet and proper sleep, so in the next session you will be able to perform better.

Cardio Activity

Once you have finished to do your warm-up, did your strength training, it is time to do some cardio.

It is useful for:

-Cardiovascular health

-Burn calories (therefore making it easier to be in a caloric deficit)

-Increase your fitness level

Here you have two options: LISS or HIIT.

-LISS stands for Low Intensity Steady State. It means doing exercises such as Cross Trainer, Walking, Jogging, Rowing machine on a low intensity for a moderate long period of time. I would do this anywhere between 15 minutes and 20 minutes at the end of the workout. Ideally you would be out of breath at the end of it.

DO NOT spend 60 minutes on them just to burn more calories and when you step out you are not even sweating…. Cardio activities help to make your body fitter, not to compensate an unhealthy diet.

-HIIT on the other hand stands for High Intensity Interval Training and consist of exercises done with high intensity with a very short rest in between. Good exercises to do the HIIT with are:

-Burpees

-Fan Bike

-Fast Running

Cool Down and Stretching

This section should last 5-10 minutes and consist of lowering down your heart rate to a baseline level (either by doing slow walking or some cycling) before doing some stretches for the muscles that have been trained.

Pick at least 3-4 positions and hold each stretch for 20-30".

TO RECAP

-Warm up part (5 to 10 minutes)

-Strength session (15 to 35 minutes)

-Pick one or two push exercises, perform each one for 3 or 4 sets of 10 reps.

-Pick one or two pull exercises, perform each one for 3 or 4 sets of 10 reps.

- Pick one or two leg exercises, perform each one for 3 or 4 sets of 10 reps.

- Pick one core exercise and perform 3 or 4 sets of 10/15 reps.

- **Cardio activity (5 to 20 minutes)**

- Pick one cardio machine and do it for 10/20 minutes. At the end of it you should be out of breath. It must be quite challenging.

- **Cool Down + Stretching (5 to 10 minutes)**

Below are examples of Full Body exercises you can do if:

-You only go three times a week in the gym.

-You are trying to lose body fat and increase muscle mass.

-You are trying to get fitter after a period of inactivity.

*No worries if you do not know the name of these exercise and how to perform them. I am going to cover everything you need to know so you will feel confident going to the gym on your own without feeling intimidated or lost.

*Also, I am giving you three examples:

-one if you just want to use resistance machine

-one if you just want to use free weights

-one if you just want to use bodyweight training (for a home workout for example!)

Obviously, you can mix up the exercises between the three categories. These are just few examples to show you how to structure it.

FULL BODY WORKOUT EXAMPLE (RESISTANCE MACHINE ONLY)

-Cross Trainer 10 minutes

-Leg Press, 4 sets of 10

-Chest Press, 4 sets of 10

-Seated Row, 4 sets of 10

-Seated Leg Curl, 4 sets of 10

-Abdominals, 3 sets of 15

-Incline Walking, 15 minutes

-Stretching, 5 minutes

FULL BODY WORKOUT EXAMPLE (FREE WEIGHTS ONLY)

-Cross Trainer 10 minutes

-BB Squat, 4 sets of 10

-DB Bench Press, 4 sets of 10

-DB Row, 4 sets of 10

-BB Hip Thrust, 4 sets of 10

-Plank Dumbbell Drag, 3 sets of 10

-Incline Walking, 15 minutes

-Stretching, 5 minutes

FULL BODY WORKOUT EXAMPLE (BODYWEIGHT ONLY)

- (Jumping Jacks and mountain Climber as a warm-up)

-Box Pistol Squat 4 sets of 10

-Push-ups, 4 sets of 10

-Inverted Rows, 4 sets of 10

-Glute Bridge, 4 sets of 10

-Plank, 3 sets of 60"

-Side Plank 2 sets each side of 30"

-Incline Walking, 15 minutes

-Stretching, 5 minutes

*This is just a random workout, sets and reps have to be adjusted to

your fitness level to make it challenging enough.

In case you really love going to the gym and you really feel better (not only physically but also in terms of mental health) this is the alternative you would do 4 days a week. It will consist of upper body, Lower Body, Upper Body, Lower Body.

For example, let's imagine you can go to the gym (or workout at home)

Monday-Upper Body

Wednesday- Lower Body

Friday- Upper Body

Saturday- Lower Body

It will allow you to work on some isolation exercises that doing full body you are probably not going to do in a Full Body Split.

UPPER BODY WORKOUT EXAMPLE

-Rowing Machine 5 minutes

-Chest Press 4 sets of 10

-Seated Row 4 sets of 10

-DB Shoulder Press 4 sets of 10

-Lat Pull Down 4 sets of 10

-Cable Bicep Curl 3 sets of 12

-Cable Triceps Pushdown 3 sets of 12

-Plank 3 set per max

LOWER BODY WORKOUT EXAMPLE

-Incline Walking 10 minutes

-Squat 4 sets of 10

-RDL 4 sets of 10

-Walking Lunges 4 sets of 10

-Hip thrust 4 sets of 10

-Leg Extension 3 sets of 12

-Seated Leg Curl 3 sets of 12

These were just some examples. As you can see in the second part of the book for each exercise there are some alternatives, so you can change them in case you cannot perform one (due to equipment limitations or other reasons).

SPECIAL OFFER: do you feel like you need an extra help and accountability for your fitness journey? Go to **avfitness99.wixsite.com** or DM me on **Instagram- avfitness99-** and see the different possibilities that you can get from Online Coaching.

PERSONALISED PLAN

Tailored 4 weeks plan based on your goals and gym frequency

-Free Zoom Consultation

-4 weeks plan

-Video Tutorial for Each Exercise

MONTHLY COACHING
**Perfect for people
serious to get fit**

-Free Zoom Consultation

-4 weeks plan

-Video Tutorial for Each
 Exercise

-Nutritional Guidelines

-Training Check 2x/weekly

-Answer to any question
 within 24 hours

ELITE COACHING
**Full accountability for
training /lifestyle**

-Free Zoom Consultation

-4 weeks personalised plan

-Video Tutorial for each exercise

-Nutritional advice

-Lifestyle advice

-Daily text for workout

-Daily text for diet/lifestyle

-24/7 Support and accountability

-2 Zoom individualized HIIT
 Workout a month

Now let's go back to the book!

*The offer might change overtime. Look at my Instagram or website to stay in touch
with the most recent updates.*

AVFITNESS99

SCAN ME

SECOND PART

There are three main categories of exercises: Resistance machines, Free Weights, and Bodyweight exercises.

For each category there are different movements:

-Pushing Exercises (chest, triceps, and shoulder)

-Pulling Exercises (for back and biceps)

-Arms Exercises

-Core Exercises

-Leg Exercises (for quadriceps, glutes, and hamstrings mainly)

For each exercise it is provided: why you should do it, how to do it (with illustrative pictures), how to progress it and regress it, the common mistakes to avoid (with illustrative pictures), the main alternatives and lastly, how would that exercise feel.

WHY

I do believe that knowing why you do a certain exercise is as important as knowing how to do it. In fact, if I tell you to do BB squat and simply instruct you, you will probably do it well. However, if I instruct you on how to perform it and tell you why it is beneficial for you (depending on

your goals, such as be more athletic, be stronger, having bigger glutes etc. etc.) you will give something more to perform it at your best.

MUSCLES WORKED

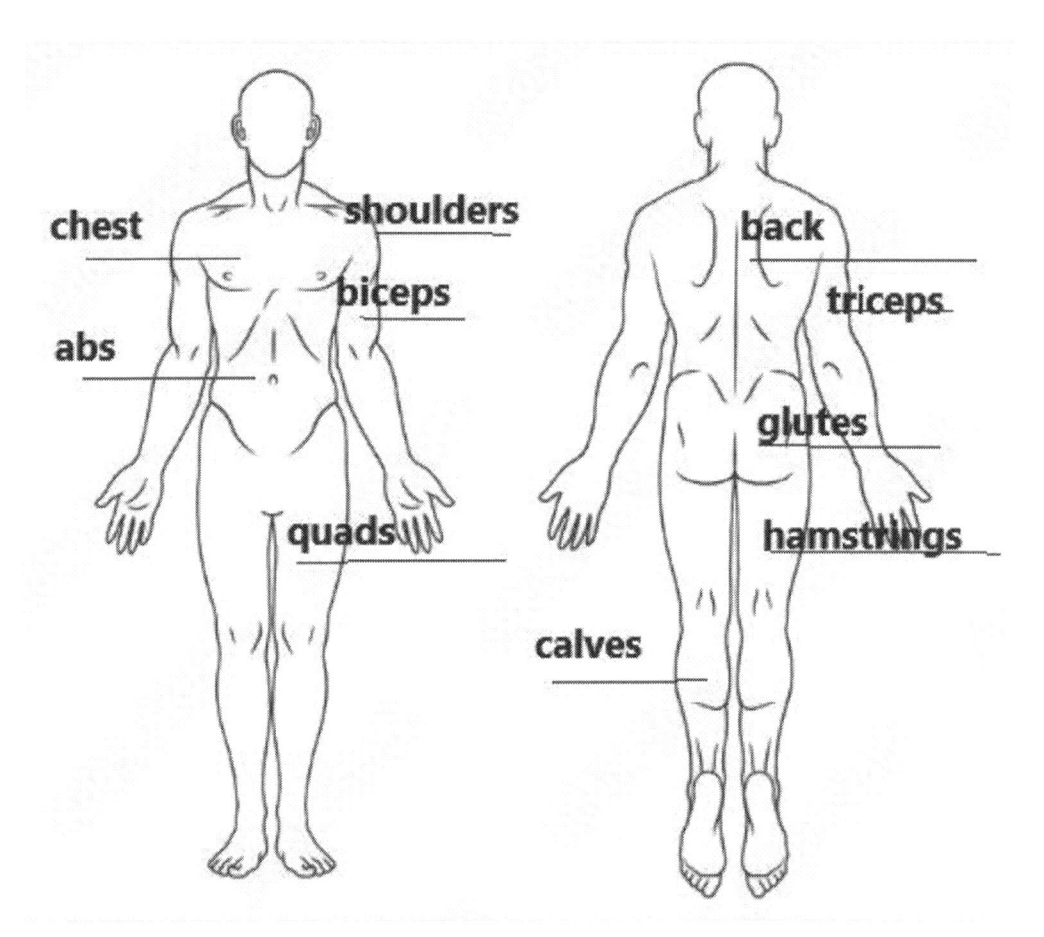

Diagram of front and back of human body with muscle labels: chest, shoulders, biceps, abs, quads (front); back, triceps, glutes, hamstrings, calves (back).

This is beneficial so you know exactly where you should be feeling it. Moreover, it will help you plan your workouts.

Note that in many free weight and bodyweight exercises some muscle act as stabilisers and have some roles in it. However, we are just going to consider the main muscle worked.

Moreover, I am going to write the muscles involved from the more involved to the less involved.

For example:

Chest Press mainly work your chest, and then there is some work done from the triceps and anterior shoulders.

Therefore, it will look like this:

Muscle worked

Chest, Triceps and Shoulder (anterior part)

HOW

How to do it is key. In fact, it is the most important thing. If you do it well with light weight you will get more benefits 8and less likelihood of injury) of doing it wrong with a heavy weight. Put your ego aside when lifting is key and ensuring that technique is perfect is the way to go.

REGRESSION/PROGRESSION

Knowing regression and progression will allow you to work the same exercise to the extent that would be challenging for you and your fitness level. Choosing a variation too easy or too difficult would decrease the effectiveness of your training.

COMMON MISTAKES TO AVOID

Being aware of the common mistakes to avoid, especially as a beginner can be extremely helpful. In fact, knowing what to do and what to avoid is key to execute an exercise properly.

ALTERNATIVES

Putting alternatives will give you more possibility of choice. Let's say that you plan to do a specific exercise, but you cannot perform it (your gym

does not have the equipment, the machine Is buys or simply you want to do something different).

By providing many alternatives the idea is to help you having a wide variety of "Plan B exercises" so you can still get an effective workout!

HOW WOULD IT FEEL?

Knowing how an exercise would feel when done right is crucial. In fact, at first you might not feel it in the muscle where you are supposed to feel. Being aware of it is a huge step for not being intimidated in the gym and on your fitness journey.

KEY RULE #1

To improve your body and fitness progressive overload and consistency are key. That means train multiple times a week and always trying to lift more, do more reps/sets and improve your technique on a regular basis.

KEY RULE #1

You should do in between 10 and 20 sets per muscle group every week. Bigger muscles, such as chest, quads and back will need less sets (10 is a good target), while smaller muscles, such as biceps, triceps and biceps can be pushed up to 20 sets.

Note: as you will see when showing the exercises, most of them works many muscles at the same time. For example, squat will work your glutes and quads at the same time (and other muscle to a lesser extent),

while push-ups will work your chest, triceps, and shoulder (and core to a lesser extent).

It means that if you are looking for general fitness and nothing specific, doing 10 sets of squats and 10 sets of pushups is more than enough to have toned and strong quads, glutes and chest, triceps, and shoulders.

Obviously, if you really want to optimize your fitness and strength level you would incorporate other exercises.

KEY RULE #1

Do not move up in weight until you OWN it.

Yes, you must strive for increasing load overtime if your technique is spot on!

That means controlling the weight in all phases of the exercise, instead of mindlessly doing reps rushed and uncontrolled to finish them.

KEY RULE #1

Stick with 2-3 exercises for each part (pushing exercise, pulling exercise and legs) for 4-6 weeks. Your goal is to get better at this. Stop changing your routine every week if you want to see progress.

KEY RULE #1

Results= Training + Sleep + Diet

Training = Hit the gym consistently and perform the exercises correctly with a progressive overload. Do your best in every session even though you feel tired or lazy. Your best that day won't be your 100%, and that's ok.

Sleep = Ideally anywhere between 7 to 9 hours. Realistically, this is difficult for many people. Aim for at least 6 hours on a consistent basis.

Diet= Ideally you would remove all the junk food, avoid eating outside your meals, increase your protein, increase daily consume of vegetables and fruit. Realistically, just try to eat a bit cleaner and healthier.

KEY RULE #1

Apply the rules below from now on, even when you do not feel like it.

*You might know already some of the rules above from reading the first part of the book, or from your own experience…anyway it is always important to keep them in mind!

Enough for the intro…. let's get started!

RESISTANCE MACHINE

This is probably the entry level for many gym-goers.

Luckily in every gym there would be plenty of this to allow you to get a full body workout even though you are not too sure what to do. Most probably there would be the name on the machine and the muscle worked.

It is easier than free weights as you need stabilization and body awareness to perform the exercise. At the same time, most of them are extremely easy to use.

This guide will show you the main machine that you can use to develop muscle in all areas of your body.

If you:

-are a skinny teenager that want to bulk up and want to start with something joint-friendly

with little or no coaching

-Are a teenager that want to lose weight but "tone up" at the same time without feeling

intimated using dumbbells and barbells

-are a man in your 40s/50s that want to take seriously your fitness but do not know when to

start

-are a woman that feel overwhelmed every time you step in the gym because everyone

knows what they are doing, and you do not have a clue

-are an elderly person that just want to get strong to recue arthritis and other potential

illnesses

This guide is for you, and these exercises will help you step up your fitness level!

UPPER BODY

-PUSH EXERCISES

Chest Press

Why

Pushing horizontally is one of the basic movement patterns of the human body.

It will work your chest, triceps, and anterior shoulder.

Muscles worked

Chest, Triceps and Shoulder (anterior part)

How

-Adjust the seat so the handles are in line with your lower chest. Do not have the handles shoulder height. In that case the elbows would flare out, and it might create shoulder pain over time.

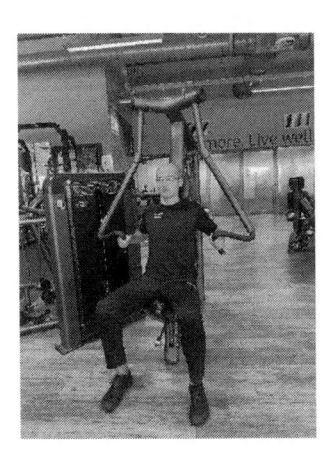

-Keep your upper back against the seat and keep your chest out throughout the movement. The only points of contact with the seat are going to be your glutes, your upper back area, and your head (slight arch on your low back is needed to protect your spine).

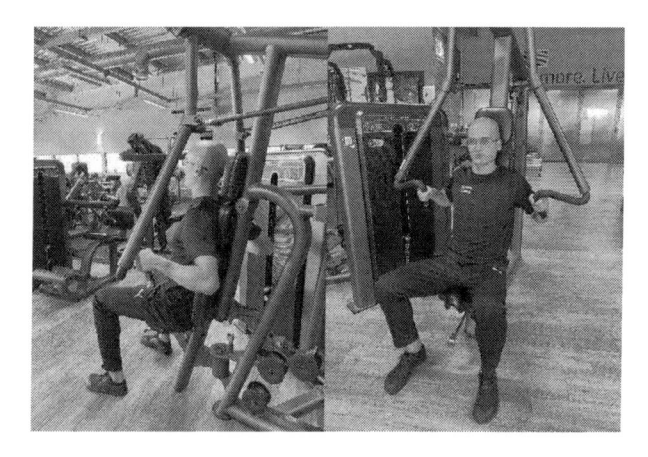

-Grab the closer handles to work more on your triceps.

-Grab the other handles to work more on your shoulder and chest.

-Push the handles in front of you and stop just before locking out the arms.

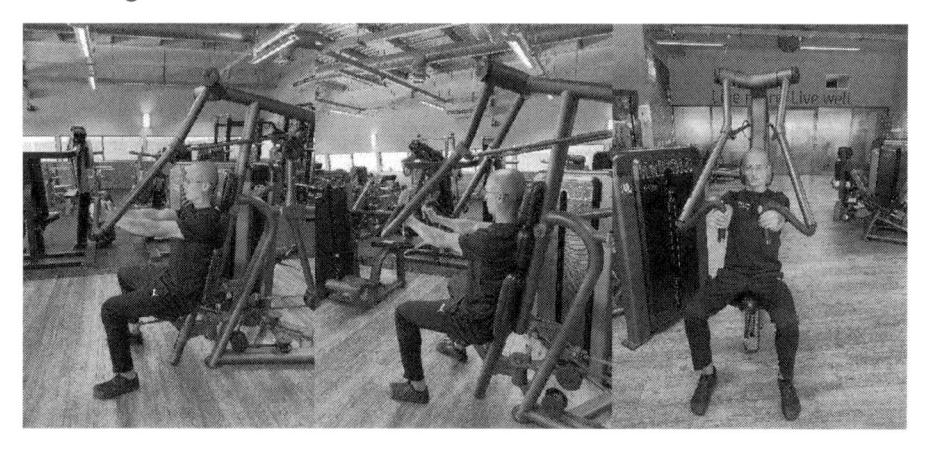

-Come back slowly to start position.

-Push again just before the weights touch each other. It should be roughly 90°.

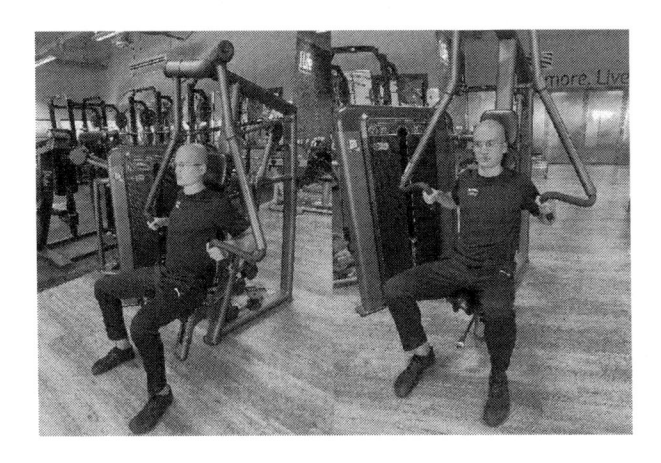

Regression/Progression

-Simply progress and regress adjusting the weight. The more weight you put, keeping your technique perfect, the better.

-Once you can do 10 comfortable reps with a given weight, I will suggest you increasing the load of 5kg (for most gym equipment it would be the next block where to insert the pin).

Common Mistakes to Avoid

-Shoulder come forward when pushing. It must be avoided as it might create shoulder pain overtime, especially with higher load.

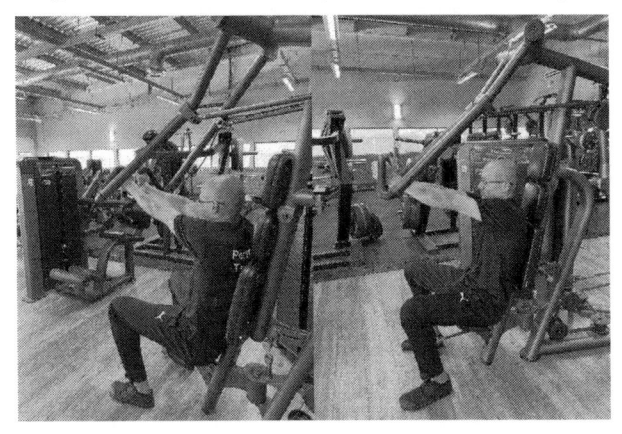

-Bouncy reps. This is not showable by photos. Make sure that the tempo of your reps is smooth and controlled. Avoid fast reps, especially if beginner and you do not master the movement yet.

-Let the weight touch and lose the tension at the bottom. It is important to keep the muscle under tension throughout the entire movement as it might lead to a better performance.

Alternatives

-DB Chest Press (page 68)

-Push-ups (page 121)

How would it feel?

If you are a beginner, you'll feel it mainly on your arms. That's' normal and it is not wrong. However, as you familiarize with this machine throughout the weeks, and making sure your chest is out during the movement, you will feel more chest activation.

Shoulder Press

Why

This is a basic vertical movement. It will work triceps and shoulders at the same time. It is easy to overload and beginner friendly.

Muscles Worked

Shoulder and Triceps

How

-Adjust the seat so that the handles are roughly in line with your shoulder.

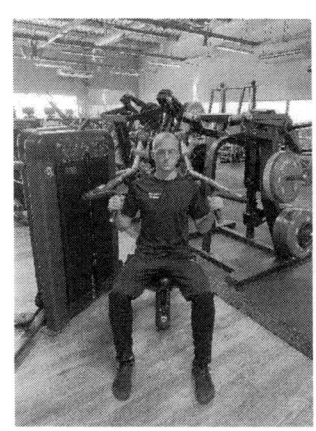

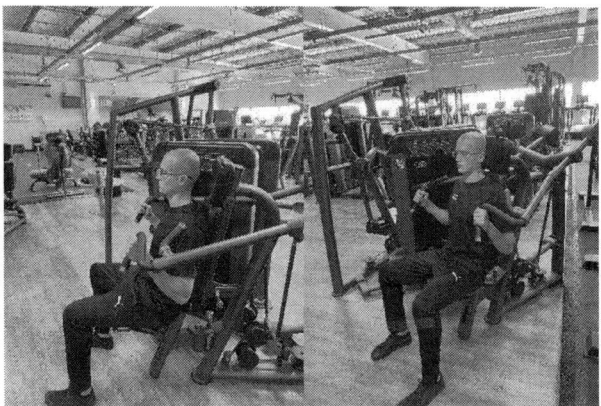

-Push the handles all the way over your head. You can lock your elbows as long as you are active in that position. It means that once you get there you will squeeze your triceps (back of the arms).

Sit comfortably and grab the handles. You can decide to have a wider grip to work more the anterior part of the shoulder. Or using a closer grip to work more on your triceps.

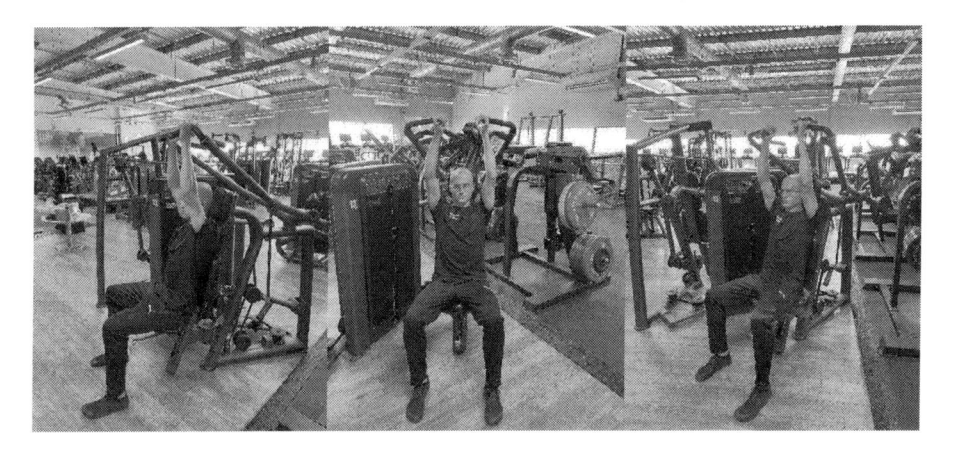

-Come back down slowly and push again before the weight touch each other. It is important to push before the weight touch each other so you keep the tension on your muscle.

Regression/Progression

-As it is a machine you will simply progress and regress adjusting the weight. Once you can do 10 reps, I would suggest you increase the load slightly.

Common Mistakes to Avoid

-Doing it too fast and rushing through the reps. Do not ego lift. Make every rep count. Performing reps in a controlled manner is key for building muscle and injury prevention.

-Shrug when you push over your head. Shoulders must be relaxed and as you push the weight up.

Alternatives

-DB Overhead Press (page 74)

-Dips (page 121)

How would it feel?

You will mainly feel it on your shoulder once you start pushing while you feel more your triceps (back of the arms) once you lock out the arms on top.

If you are a beginner, it might be that after just a few reps you feel your muscle burning. If that is the case, I would suggest you focusing on your breathing (inhaling on the way down

and exhaling when you push the handles up). This would allow you to give more oxygen to the muscle and therefore feel stronger for longer.

Pec Fly Machine

Why

Although this is not necessarily a pushing movement; we can put it in this category as it works primarily your chest. It is a good exercise to learn how to work your chest muscle, which is especially important for many pushing exercise (pushups, bench press, dips etc. etc.).

It will also work your biceps and, considering the nature of the movement, will work on your posture too.

Muscle worked

Chest and Biceps (to a much lesser degree)

How

-Grab the handles and always keep your arms straight (a minor bend at the elbows is allowed, but no more than that).

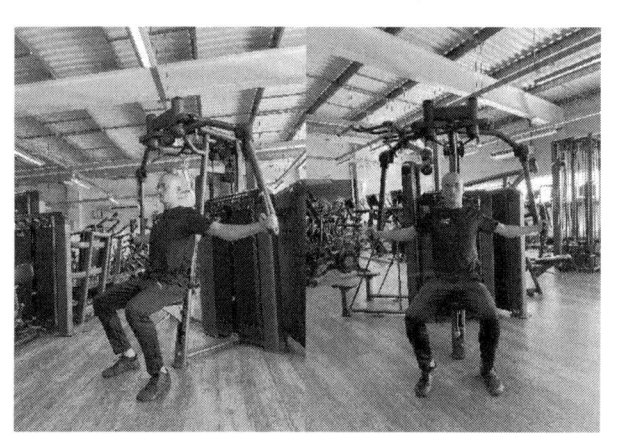

-Make sure that your palms are in line with your chest and not with your shoulders (it might create shoulder pain).

-While always keeping your chest out and arms straight, push the handles together.

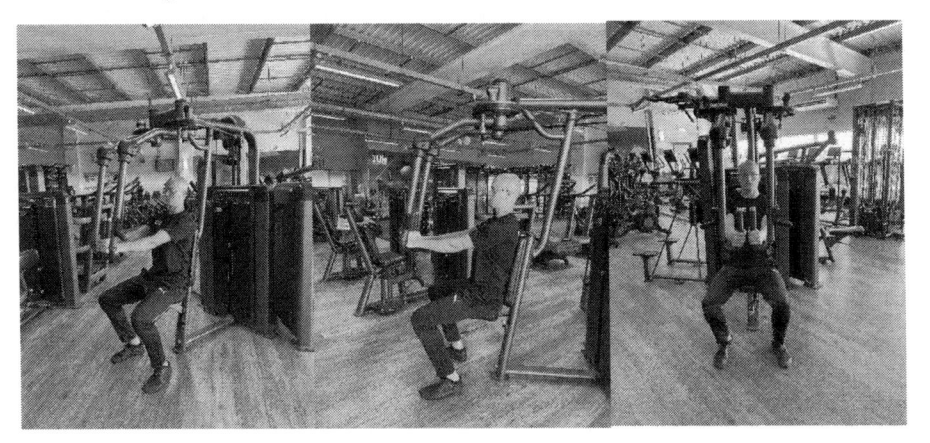

-Hold them for a second and focus on squeezing your chest.

-Come back to starting position in a slow and controlled manner and go again.

Regression/Progression

-You simply adjust the load based on your strength level. As a rule, once you can do 10 reps with a given weight quite comfortably, I would suggest you increase the load slightly.

-Moreover, in this machine you can increase or decrease the range of motion. More range of motion will result in more muscle as well as healthier pcs. It would have a carryover on your posture (avoid hunching).

Common Mistakes to Avoid

As mentioned before:

-Do not bend your elbow when performing it otherwise you will work your biceps and anterior shoulder rather than your chest)

-Do not have the handles in line with your shoulders. Adjust the seat as the handles are in line with your mid chest.

Alternatives

-DB Fly (page 72)

-Chest Flyes at Cable Machine (page 36)

How would it feel?

You will feel a good stretch to start the movement. Then, throughout the movement you will probably feel the lateral side of your chest working. Lastly, when the handles are in contact you will feel the area in the middle of your chest do most of the work. If, when closing the handle together, you do not feel it there, but you feel it more on your arms, revisit your technique by focusing on the teaching points above.

Chest Flyes at Cable Machine

Why

It is a great exercise to work your chest and isolate it in ways that normal presses do not do. However, make sure to learn the right technique as for many people the anterior part of the shoulder takes over!

If done right, this exercise will work your stretch under load in a stretched position. This is key for your posture. In fact, many chest exercises do not work your chest in this deep range of motion, leaving gains on the table.

Muscle Worked

Chest and Biceps (to a much lesser degree)

How

-Grab on handle at the time.

-Prior performing the movement (this is the KEY) retract and push down your shoulder blades. By doing that you will create the perfect set up for chest activation. Keep it this way throughout the movement

PS: by doing this you will inevitably turn your arm slightly outward.

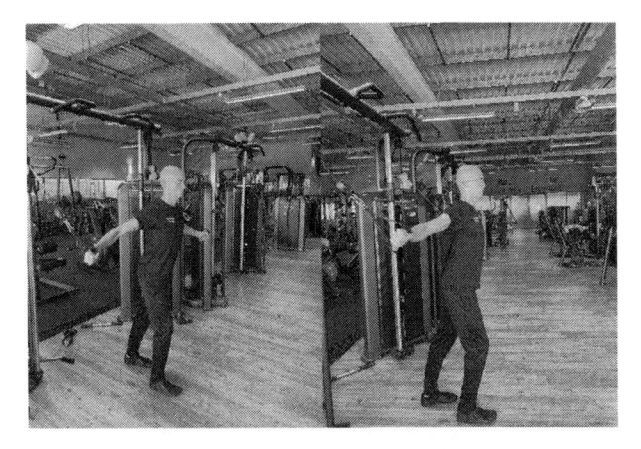

-From starting position bring your arms together. Your arms should be almost straight throughout the movement. Make sure to bring your elbows/biceps together rather than your

hands (by doing this you will avoid your biceps and anterior shoulders to take over). This will allow maximal chest contraction.

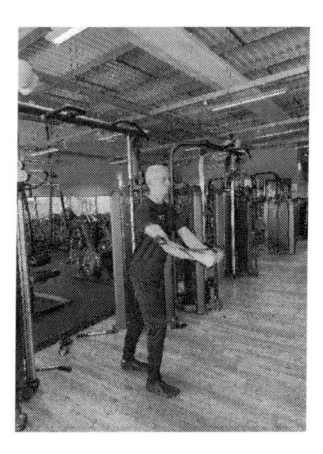

-Squeeze on top of the movement for half a second.

-Then go back slowly into starting position keeping your chest out. This will allow your chest to be completely stretched, enhancing his strength throughout a long range of motion.

Note: make sure to keep your initial set up

throughout the movement!

Regression/Progression

-Start with a light weight and get used to right technique with high reps (even over 15 per sets).

-Slowly increase the weight. However, progression in this exercise is more on time under tension and reps (and other advanced techniques) rather than lifting heavy weight. This exercise should be an accessory that you perform towards the end of the training. At the start of your training focus on other exercise such as Dips, Bench Press, Overhead Press, and other compound movements.

Common Mistakes to Avoid

-Too much weight. Avoid this at all costs. Unfortunately, it is quite common to see people "ego lift" this movement. Do not be one of them.

-Rolling your shoulders forward. This will let the shoulders do most of the work.

Alternatives

-DB Flys (page 72)

-Pec Flyes (page 33)

How would it feel?

If done right, you will feel a strong activation on your chest. This exercise allows you really to stretch and squeeze your chest muscle. Take advantage of it if you want to build a strong and big chest. Not may exercises provide those two movements for your chest as good as chest flies at the cable machine does. I would also suggest you squeeze your lats when performing the movement. By doing that you will be automatically deactivate your shoulders from doing most of the work

SPECIAL OFFER: do you feel like you need an extra help and accountability for your fitness journey? Go to **avfitness99.wixsite.com** or DM me on **Instagram- avfitness99-** and see the different possibilities that you can get from Online Coaching.

PERSONALISED PLAN

Tailored 4 weeks plan based on your goals and gym frequency

-Free Zoom Consultation

-4 weeks plan

-Video Tutorial for Each Exercise

MONTHLY COACHING
Perfect for people serious to get fit

- Free Zoom Consultation

- 4 weeks plan

- Video Tutorial for Each Exercise

- Nutritional Guidelines

- Training Check 2x/weekly

- Answer to any question within 24 hours

ELITE COACHING
Full accountability for training /lifestyle

- Free Zoom Consultation

- 4 weeks personalised plan

- Video Tutorial for each exercise

- Nutritional advice

- Lifestyle advice

- Daily text for workout

- Daily text for diet/lifestyle

- 24/7 Support and accountability

- 2 Zoom individualized HIIT Workout a month

Now let's go back to the book!

***The offer might change overtime. Look at my Instagram or website to stay in touch**

with the most recent updates.

AVFITNESS99

SCAN ME

-PULL EXERCISES

Seated Row

Why

This is a great pulling exercise that is easy to perform and work many muscles in your back as well as biceps. Moreover, since nowadays we spent many times sitting and hunching our back, exercises of pulling will help to improve your posture.

Muscles Worked

Back, Biceps and Shoulder (posterior part)

How

-Grab the handle with a neutral grip and sit with knees slightly bent.

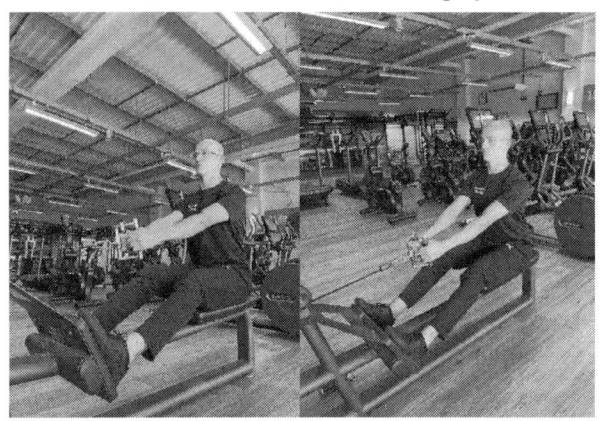

-Keep your chest up and shoulders down and relaxed throughout the movement.

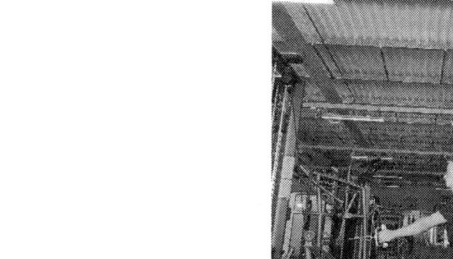

-Pull the handle towards your belly button.

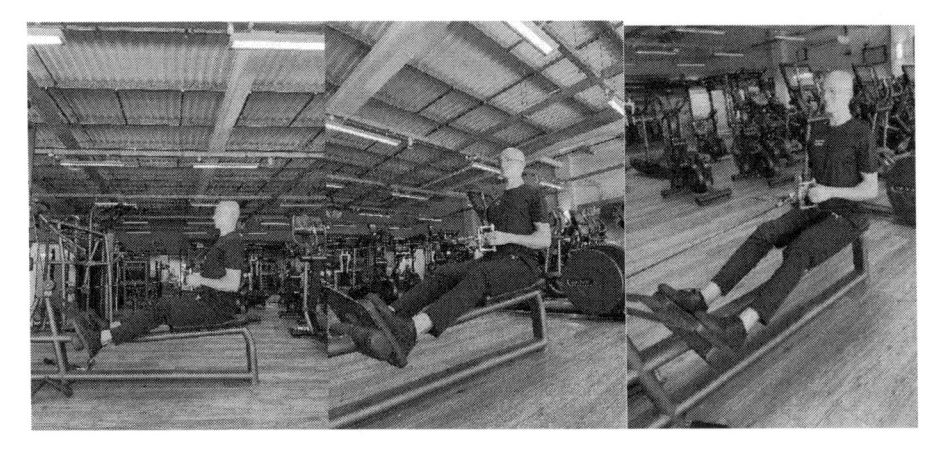

-Control the eccentric part (the one in which the handle is going away from you).

Regression/Progression

As the previous exercises, being a machine the way in which you progress or regress it is simply by adjusting the load. A good idea would be increasing the load once 10 reps with a given weight are done comfortably.

Common Mistakes to Avoid

-Going through the motion and treat this exercise as a rowing machine (page xx). To avoid this, make sure just to keep your body straight.

-Rounding your back and coming with your shoulders forward. To avoid this, make sure to keep your chest up and shoulders back and down.

Alternatives

-DB Row (page 83)

-Inverted Row (page 129)

How would it feel?

You should feel your back muscle squeezing as you pull the handle towards you. The first few times is likely that you will mainly (or only) feel on your arms. However, you should be focusing on contracting the muscle around your shoulder blades as you pull, and you will eventually feel your back working.

Lat Pulldown

Why

Seated Row is a good horizontal pulling movement. However, as we previously mentioned one horizontal and one vertical pull, we now must mention a vertical pull. It works your back and biceps.

Muscles Worked

Back and Biceps

How

-Grab the handles just where it curves and put your thumb around for a close grip.

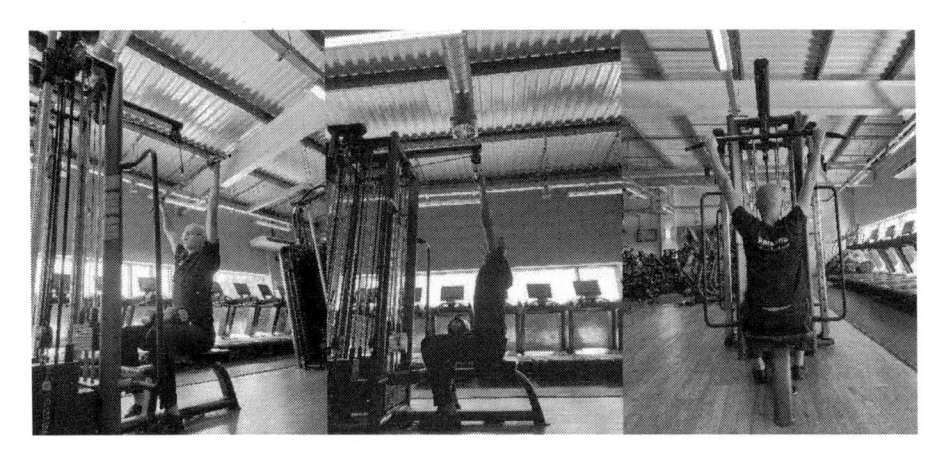

-Sit with the pad just above your thigs.

-Arch your upper back slightly to lift your chest up.

-Pull the bar towards your lower chest.

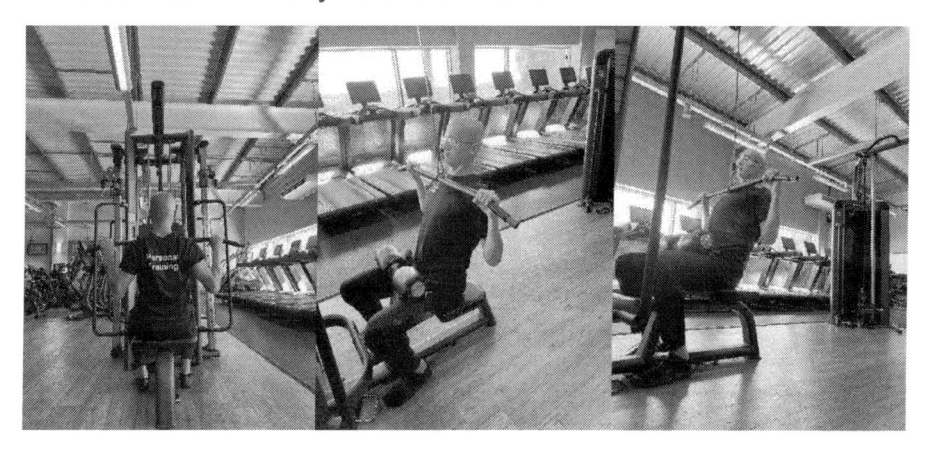

-Go back into starting position controlling the movement.

Regression/Progression

Increase and decrease the weight accordingly. Once you can do 10 reps comfortably, I would increase weight.

Common Mistakes to Avoid

-Bringing the bar too low. This would recruit other muscle and might also be uncomfortable for your shoulders.

-Staying flat with your back. By staying completely flat under the bar you will limit the back activation tremendously. Avoid this by slightly leaning backwards.

-Unbalanced grip making the exercise uncomfortable. One hand way closer than the other hand.

-Setting the pad too low. As shown above, the pad should rest on your thigs.

Alternatives

-DB Pullover (page 87)

-Chin-ups (page 126)

How would it feel?

At first you might struggle a bit with the movement, and you will feel the arms doing most of the work. However, if you stick with it for a few weeks and keep in mind the teaching points given, you will feel your back muscle pulling the bar, and contracting every time you pull the bar towards you.

CORE EXERCISES

Abdominals Machine

Why

Your abdominal muscles are arguably one of the most important muscles when it comes to strength and movement. In fact, we engage our abs in any movement we perform, inside or outside the gym. The degree of strength of your abs determines the ability to perform your daily life activities. This exercise is easy to learn, and anyone can do it to start.

Muscles Worked

Abs

How

-Select the desired load.

-Sit down and grab the handles.

-Put the pad against the area between your chest and shoulders.

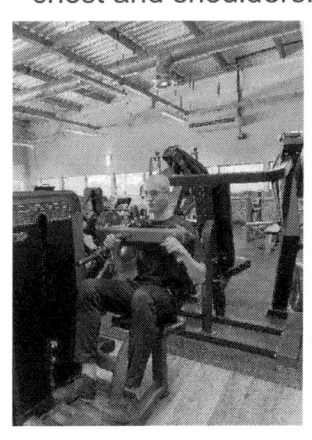

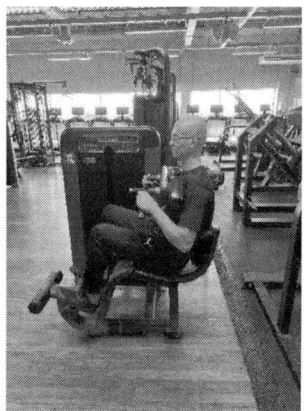

-Push the pad down with your chest (imagine doing a crunch).

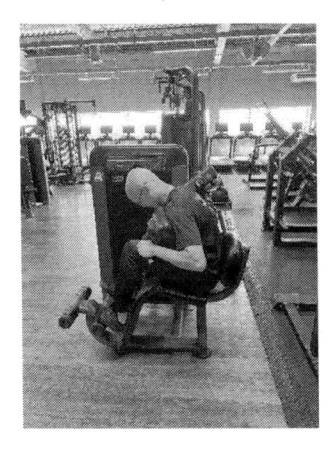

-Hold at the bottom for half a second and go back up slowly.

-Before the weight touches, push the pad down again.

Regression/Progression

-Simply decrease or increase the weight. For this exercise I would do anywhere between 12 and 20 reps per set. I would personally stay more between 12-15 but it is more of a personal choice.

Common Mistakes to Avoid

-Losing the tension at the top. As many machines, you should always keep the tension on your muscle. In fact, the weight must never touch each other during a set.

-Pushing with your hands. You should push the pad down with your chest. By doing so, you will activate your abs.

How would it feel?

Just make sure you do not feel it on your low back. Ideally you would feel it entirely on your abs. If that is not the case, try to lower down the intensity and/or do less reps. If you still feel it on your lower back (unlikely) I would suggest you not to perform this exercise for a while.

ARMS EXERCISES
Cable Bicep Curl

Why

It is a good exercise for your biceps. By doing this at the cable machine, you will have less pressure on your elbow tendon than doing this exercise with dumbbells. It makes this exercise joint-friendly and effective for muscle growth.

Muscles Worked

Biceps

How

-Put the cable attachment as low as possible.

-Grab the bar with an underhand grip (simply means palms facing you). Make sure to really squeeze the handle. This is often overlooked but it is extremely important to perform this exercise effectively.

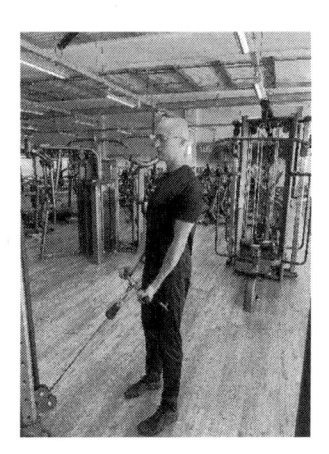

-Keep your elbows tucked in the whole time during the execution.

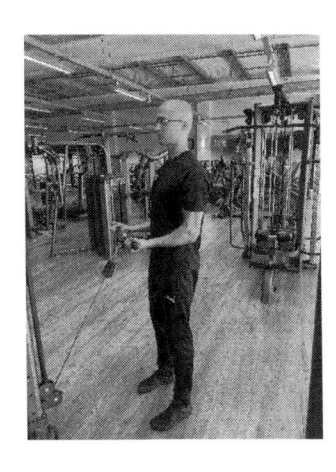

-Push the bar up until your wrist almost touches your shoulder. Do it in a very slow and controlled manner. Making the repetitions fast and rushed do not make them more effective.

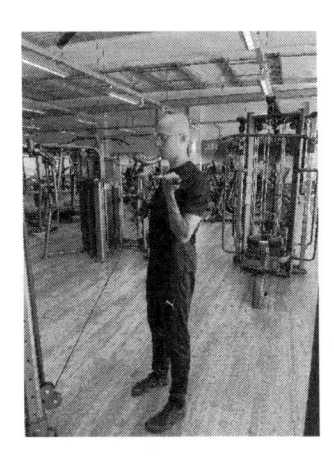

-Come back down and fully stretch your arms. Make sure to have your arms straight. It will allow not only the muscle to lengthen but also the connective tissue aka tendons and ligaments (it is good for training longevity).

-Push the bar up again and fully squeeze for 1 second on top of the movement.

Regression/Progression

-You can simply adjust the load of this exercise. I would not go below 10 reps when performing this exercise. being an accessory exercise that only work the bicep, I would suggest you use it towards the end of your training and performing 10/15 reps per set.

Common Mistakes to Avoid

-Drive your elbow in front of you. It is a common mistake that people do to lift more weight. However, by doing that you do not work your biceps but put less pressure on your anterior part of the shoulder and on your joints.

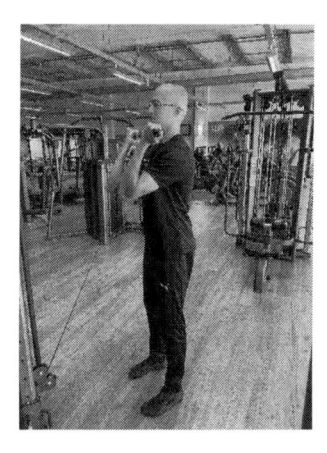

-Not closing the reps. Bring the bar all the way up is necessary to fully squeeze the bicep on top and fully gain the benefit of this exercise.

How would it feel?

When you first push you will feel a stretch on your arms. The first part is easy. The middle range is the most difficult (here is important to keep your elbows still"). At the end of the movement make sure to squeeze your biceps for maximal growth.

Just make sure to pick a weight that is light enough to really feel your bicep working. In fact, this is not the type of exercise where you aim to lift more weight, but to do more reps and really feel it in your muscle.

Cable Triceps Pushdown

Why

This is a good exercise to work your arms. If you are a guy that is looking to have bigger arms or a woman that is looking to "tone up" her arms, this exercise is a good accessory to your training. Moreover, it might be helpful in case your arms are the weakest link in some other exercises. In fact, especially for beginners, improving your strength in this exercise might facilitate the execution of pushups.

Muscles Worked

Triceps

How

-Use the cable machine and put the attachment as high as possible.

-Step back and grab the rope from its extremities.

-keep your elbows tucked to the side. It is not going to move during the exercise.

-Push the rope down and fully extend your arm at the bottom.

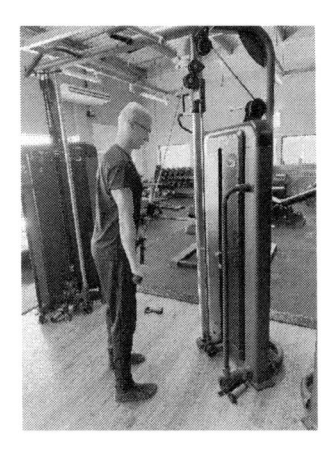

-Come back up to 90°, and then push down again.

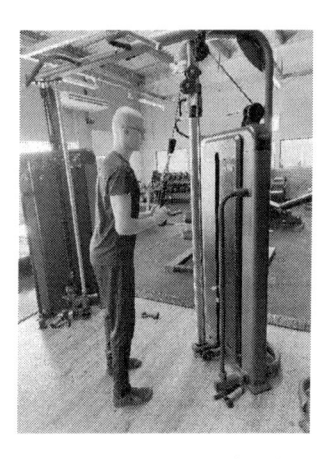

*Also, you can do the same exercise using different tool such as the v-bar or a straight bar. With the rope, however, you can maximise your range of motion, so I would suggest using that one.

Regression/Progression

-Simply increase or decrease the weight. As for the Cable Bicep Curl, I would stay in between 10 and 15 reps.

Common Mistakes to Avoid

-Twisting wrist out. By doing so, you might think you get more range of motion aka more work for your triceps. That's not how it works unfortunately. By twisting your wrist out at the bottom of the movement you are putting excessive pressure on your wrist. Once you fully extend at the bottom you already work your triceps at max contraction

How would it feel?

To make the most out of it, this is an isolation exercise. Therefore, you want your triceps to be the only thing that is working. You would feel constant pressure on your triceps.

LOWER BODY EXERCISES

Leg press

Why

This is an easy exercise to do that works many muscles at the same time. Anyone can do it (unless major knee pain or other conditions are present. You can adjust the range of motion based on your mobility level, and you can start with very ow weight.

Muscles Worked

Quads and Glutes

How

-Adjust the handles according to your mobility (Ideally you should go as close as possible to the platform.

-Put your feet hip width apart in the middle of the platform with your toes pointing up. Then, grab the handles.

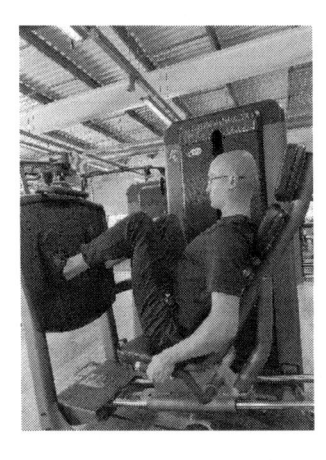

-Push with your feet until your legs are just slightly bent (do not lock your knees!)

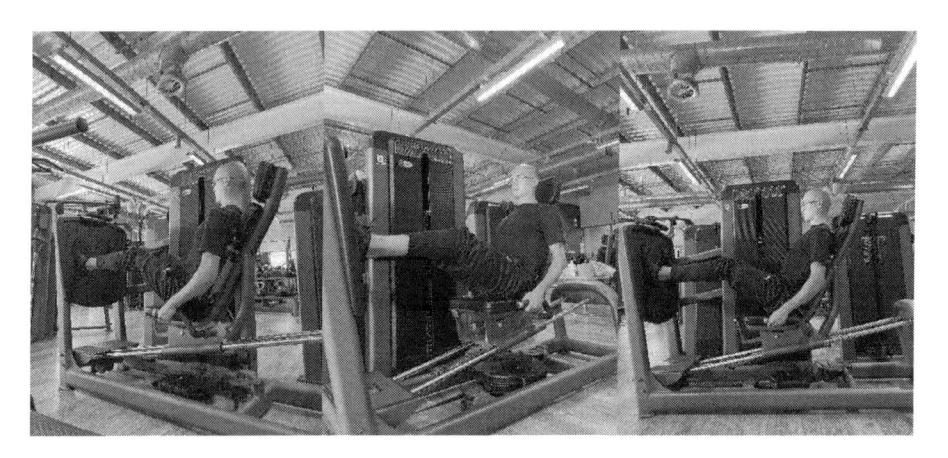

-Come back slowly down and push up just before the weight touch each other.

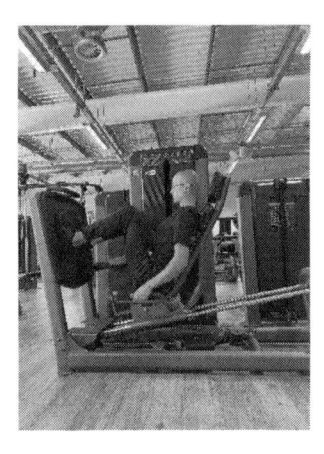

Regression/Progression

Being a resistance machine, you adjust the intensity by changing the load. Once you can comfortably do 8/10 reps it is time to increase it.

Common Mistakes to Avoid

-Caving in your knees as you push.

-Lift your toes while pushing.

-Lock out the knee.

-Keep your hands on your thighs while pushing.

Alternatives

-BB Squat (page 103)

-DB Lunges (page 113)

-Box Pistol Squat (page 136)

-Bulgarian Split Squat (page 138)

How would It feel?

This is a machine that everyone can do perfectly from the start. You will immediately feel your legs working where it is supposed to be felt. Only limitations might be for overweight people and/or people with constant knee pain. In that case I would still try to do it but with lighter load and keeping the range of motion very short to start with.

Lying Leg Curl

Why

This is an exercise that will work your hamstring in knee flexion. It is an effective exercise for people new to the gym as it is easy to learn as well as effective for more experienced gym-goers. In fact, people that have been training for years tend to work their posterior chain with exercises such as Hip Thrust, Deadlift and RDL that are hip dominant. Lying Leg curl, as well as the seated version, target the hamstring by flexing the knee.

Muscles Worked

Hamstrings (back or your leg) and Calves (to a much lesser degree)

How

-Lay down with chest on the bench and grab the handles underneath it.

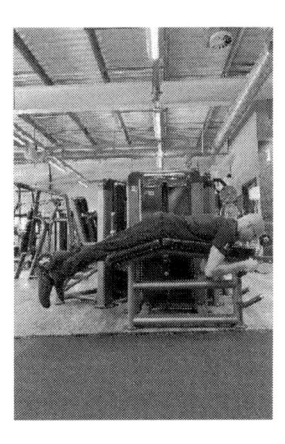

-Adjust the pad so it is just above the ankle (it should be on your Achilles tendon).

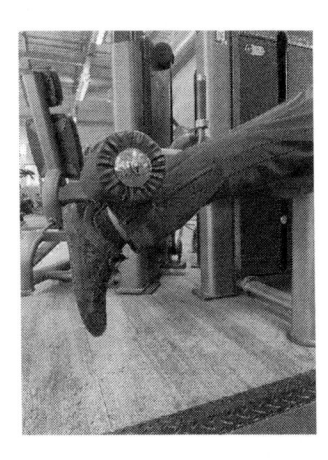

-Knees are in line with the pivot joint.

-From that position push the pad up and toward your glutes. How far? Find your end range where past that you do not feel any more hamstring activation (for most people is just after the pad is vertical to the floor.

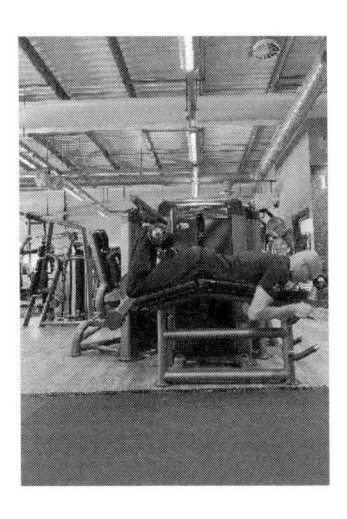

-Once you can no longer push the pad, hold the greatest degree of tension for you, and slowly come back down into starting position.

-Repeat the exercise for the desired reps.

These above is the basic version to perform this exercise. However, if you really want to get the best out of it, follow these tips below:

1- Most people do it with their foot in a dorsiflexion position (toes up). This will make you to lift more weight as you not only will work your hamstrings but also your calves will help you. To get the most out of it I suggest you stay in plantarflexion (toes down). By doing this your calves will be already contracted so most of the work will be on the hamstrings. You will lift less weight, but the exercise will be more effective.

2- Then, how far are your feet from each other? If they are hip width apart, you will be able to lift more weight. However, if you have your feet and consequently your legs closer, you will be able to feel your hamstring squeeze more, leading them to quicker growth.

3- By having your toes pointing inside, you will work more the inside of your hamstrings, while having your toes out will engage more the outer part of the hamstrings.

I would say that having your feet close with your toes pointed down and slightly in is the best set up for this exercise.

Lastly, when performing this exercise and avoid any low back discomfort you must make the pelvic area very stable. How can you do that?

-Squeeze the glutes (mild contraction is ok).

-Bring pelvis into the pad.

-Pull your upper body very tight on the pad.

These tips should help to avoid possible low back discomfort when performing the exercise as well as maximise your hamstrings" work.

Regression/Progression

-Simply increase or decrease the weight. Once you feel comfortable doing 10/12 reps with a given weight, it is time to add more load. If you do not feel comfortable putting more load you can simply make every rep slower and longer as to increase the time under tension.

Common Mistakes to Avoid

-Having the pad too high or too low. Having it lo low on your foot will make it uncomfortable as it would slide as soon as you push it up. On the other hand, having it too high close to your knee will inhibit the hamstring activation and decrease the range of motion.

-Do not bounce back from the bottom. This is quite common as it comes naturally. In fact, by doing this you will feel stronger and being able to do more reps and lift more weights (this is due to the work on the calves other than the hamstrings). However, to make this exercise as effective as possible try to hold one second at the bottom, and then come back up without using any momentum.

Alternatives

-Seated Leg Curl (page 62)

-Nordic Curl (page 159)

-Stability Ball Leg Curl (page 143)

How would it feel?

As you push the pad up you will feel your hamstring contracting (and a bit your calves). As you come down you will feel your hamstring stretching. That is very important to go down slowly to really work them and let them get stronger.

Seated Leg Curl

Why

Leg press is a great exercise but do not work your hamstring. That is why doing Leg Curl is important to avoid muscle imbalances.

Muscles Worked

Hamstrings and Calves (to a much lesser degree)

How

-Sit comfortably. For most people, the back of the knee should be in line with the hand of the seat, but this can vary person to person.

-Select the weight and grab the handle.

-Put your feet over the pad.

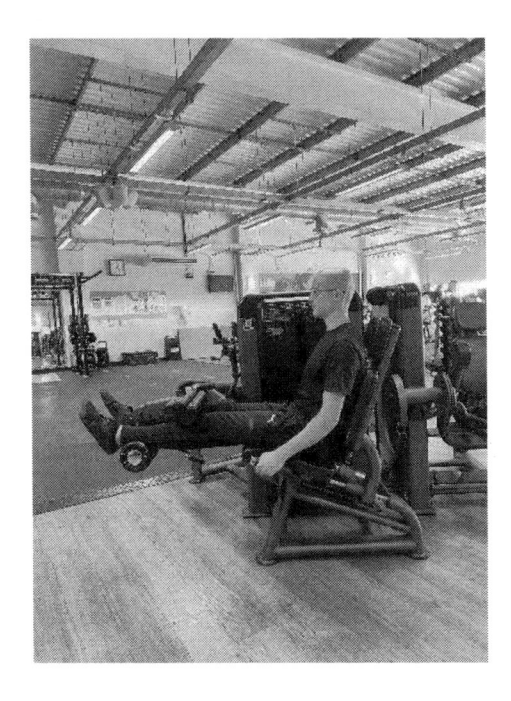

-Push the pad all the way down and hold half a second.

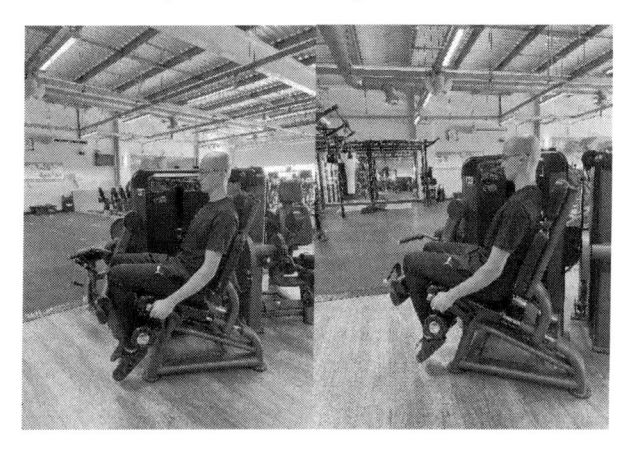

-Come back up and push the pad again before the weight touches.

*All the tips about feet positioning mentioned in the Lying Leg Curl works also for this exercise.

Regression/Progression

You can simply progress it by adjusting the weight. Once you can do 10 reps with a given weight comfortably, it is probably time to add more load.

Common Mistakes to Avoid

-Keeping the range of motion to short. If so, you should consider lower down the load.

-Bouncing the repetition, with no control (it is not possible to show it with an image, but it is important to hold at the bottom, and then come back up. Bouncing the repetitions and make them faster will not benefit you at all.)

-Come forward with your glutes while doing it.

Alternatives

-BB RDL (page 110)

-Glute Bridge (page 140)

-Nordic Curl (page 159)

How would it feel?

In this one you should feel after 3/4 reps the muscle above the back of the knee working immediately. In some cases, you might feel your calves as well. That is completely normal, and if your calves do not take over the movement there is nothing wrong.

Instead, if you feel your calves doing most of the work, you might consider pointing your toes forward when doing the exercise. By doing this you voluntarily contract your calves, and so, they will not assist as much when doing the reps.

Leg Extension

Why

While Leg Curl works the hamstrings directly, the Leg Extension works the quads (the Leg Press, as showed, works them already, but not as much. It is an incredibly good exercise for both beginners and advanced. For beginners it is good to learn how to properly extend the knee and activate your quadriceps. It is especially true for the teardrop muscle just above the knee, the VMO. For advanced is a great exercise for hypertrophy reason and as an accessory of exercises like Squats or Lunges.

Muscles Worked

Quads

How

-Sit comfortably and grab the handles.

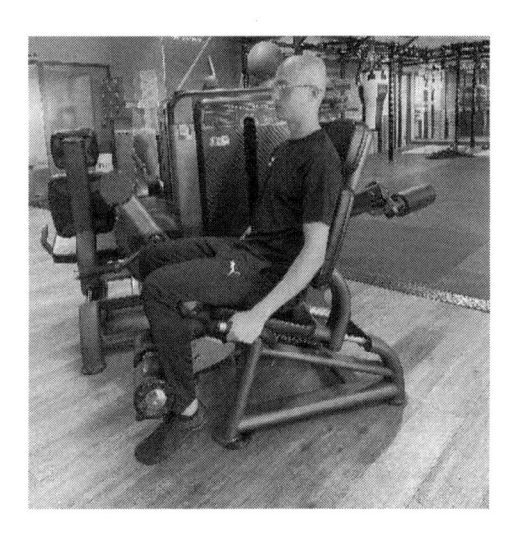

-The back of the knee should be in line with the end of the seat.

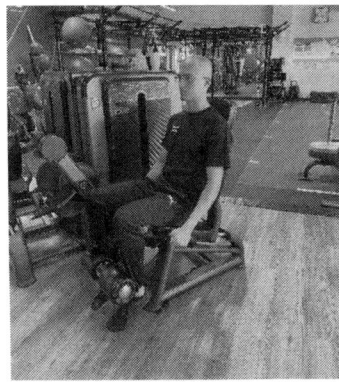

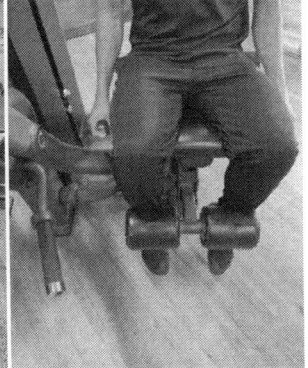

-Push the pad up and stop just before locking out your knees.

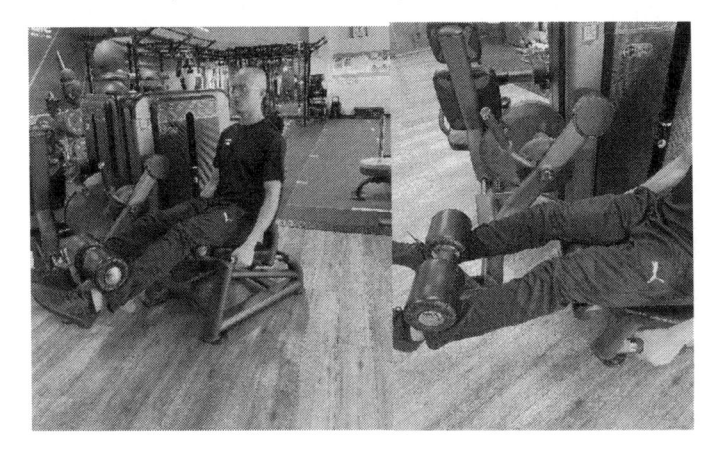

-Go down slowly and push back up just before the weights touch each other.

Regression/Progression

You simply regress it or progress it by changing the load. Once you can do 10 reps, it is probably time to challenge yourself with a higher load.

Common Mistakes to Avoid

- Bouncing the repetitions (this is a mistake that many people do unfortunately. It is not only ineffective for your muscles but also can be harmful for your knees!).

-Locking out on top. To clarify, there is some debate about this. I would not suggest you do it as it puts lots of pressure on your tendons and ligaments around your knees. On the other hand, it allows you to contract more your quads, therefore enhancing your performance.

Personally, the risk outweighs the benefit (for most people), and so I would avoid locking out the knee.

-Not having knees in line with the end of the seat in the set-up position.

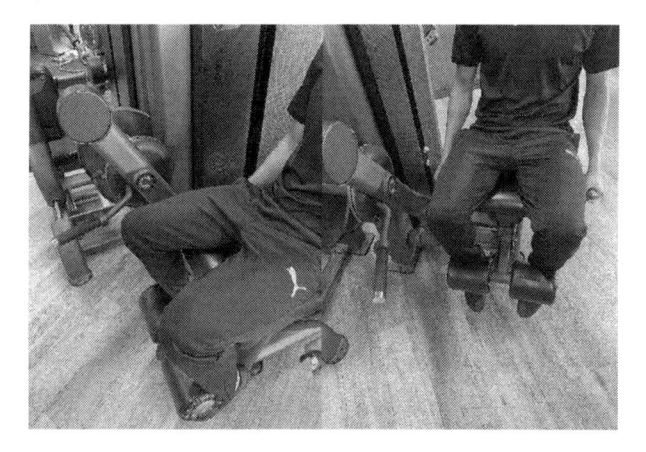

As you can see, knees are not in contact with the seat, making the exercise less effective and more dangerous for your knee's health.

Alternatives

-Reverse Nordic Curl (page 153)

How would it feel?

When you do leg extension, it is quite common to feel a burning sensation on your quads just after a few reps. That is key form muscle growing (and muscle "toning" as many gym-goers would define it).

FREE WEIGHTS

The next step in your fitness journey would be to use free weights. In fact, free weights are arguably better than resistance machine for:

-More muscle control and stabilization needed

-Ability to overload or work unilaterally effectively

-Easier to plan a workout (with a single dumbbell you can potentially do a full body workout rather than needing plenty of machines)

However, if you are not onto weights and you "just want to stay fit and toned" and changing from machine to weights will put you off from your training habits, feel free not to use them.

Personally, I think that free weights, meaning barbells and dumbbells, are a superior exercise that has an enormous carryover on any sport or daily life activities.

I would say that resistance machines are a good starting point, and if you are serious about your fitness, you must be willing to give to these exercises a shot

Here there are the basic exercises you can do that will give you tons of results if you are consistent with them and gradually overload them.

UPPER BODY

-PUSH

DB Chest Press

Why

Using dumbbells will allow you to get more range of motion as well as avoiding too much pressure on your joints (especially shoulder and wrist). Moreover, the big stretch on your chest will enhance not only the muscle to get stronger but it helps to strengthen the connective tissue (tendons, ligaments, and fascia) to be more resilient in long range of motion).

Muscles Worked

Chest, Triceps and Shoulder (anterior part)

How

-Grab two dumbbells and sit on a flat bench.

-Lay down and bring your dumbbells close you your chest.

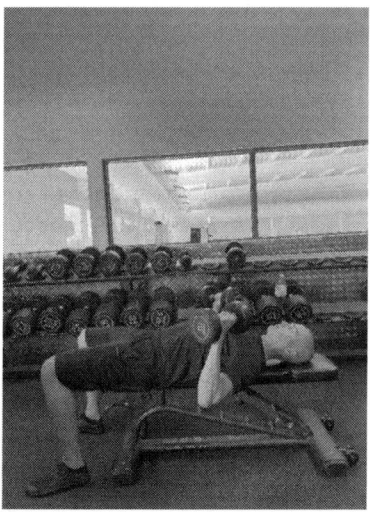

-Push the dumbbells up over your chest.

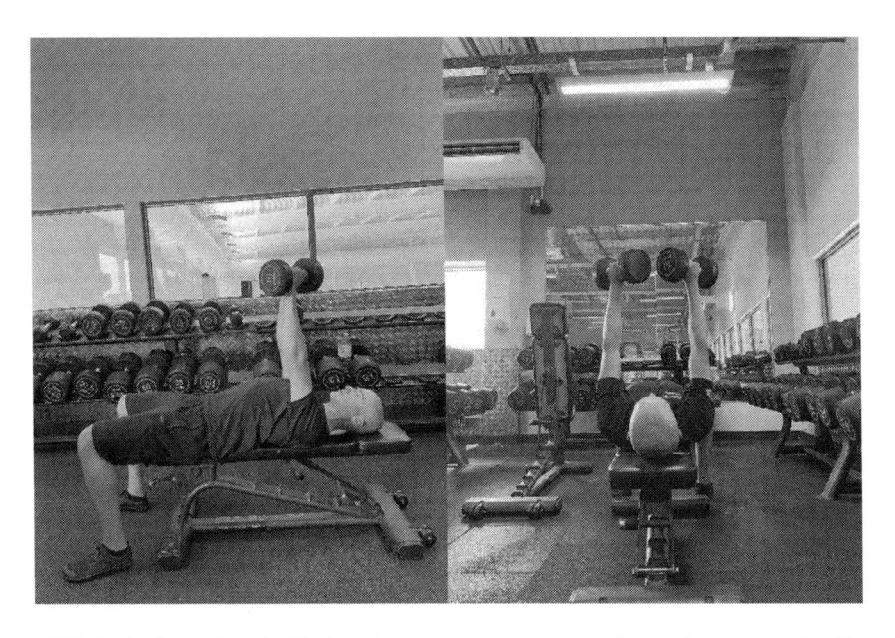

*This is just the initial set-up, now we see how to execute it.

-Bring the dumbbells down next to your chest. Let's control the way down. Perform in 2/3 seconds.

-Hold at the bottom for one second (do not bounce back using momentum!).

-Push the dumbbells back up keeping your chest out. At the end of the movement the dumbbells should be close together.

Regression/Progression

You can regress it and progress it by changing the load. You cans tart this exercise with dumbbells as low as 2.5kg! and progress up to 50kg (I have never seen anyone doing DB Chest Press with 50kg, so you can be the first one with patience and consistency!).

Common Mistakes to Avoid

-Not closing the dumbbells on top.

-Push your shoulders forwards (your chest should be out and high all the time)

Alternatives

-Chest Press (page 68)

-Push-ups (page 121)

*You can also do it inclined. The teaching pints are the same, but you are just going to incline the bench of 30/45° as to work more your upper chest.

How would it feel?

You will feel it on your triceps and chest mainly. At the bottom range, your chest and shoulders will do most of the work, while to close the dumbbells together you will feel it more on your arms.

DB FLYS

Why

This exercise is fantastic to work your chest in a stretched position that you can get when doing pushups or bench press. By working your chest in a stretched position, you will also improve your posture. In fact, this exercise will help to avoid that hunch position that you might see in some gyms. Moreover, there is no need to use heavy weight to perform it.

Muscles Worked

Chest

How

-Lay down on a bench and grab two dumbbells.

-Start by having the dumbbells just over your chest.

-From there lower down until your arms are parallel to the ground.

-Push back up into starting position while keeping your chest out.

Bonus tip. Focus on having your elbows coming closer to each other on the way up rather than your hands. It will enhance your chest activation.

Regression/Progression

-You can start by using light dumbbells to make sure the technique is on point. Then, when you feel comfortable, you will use heavier ones.

-At first you might limit the range of motion, and gradually build up to the max you can do.

Common Mistakes to Avoid

-Improper extension of your arms. At the bottom position, your elbows should be lightly bent. If you keep your arms straight, you will put excessive pressure on your shoulder joint.

(Note: there is not a thing such as too much pressure. In this guideline I am generalizing. For 99% of the people having your arms straight in that position might cause shoulder pain as the connective tissue around that area are not used to be stretched under load).

-Do not extend too far. It is good to feel a mild stretch on your chest but do not hyper extend too far. As a rule, I would say that having your arms parallel to the ground is a good goal for almost everyone.

Alternatives

-Pec. Fly machine (page 33)

How would it feel?

For more chest activation, at the end of the movement try to squeeze your elbows together. By doing that you will feel the inner part of your chest working a lot more. Instead, if you squeeze your hands together, you will feel it more on your biceps (that is not what you want).

DB Overhead Press

Why

Using dumbbells allow more range of motion than using resistance machine or barbells as well as requiring more control and stabilization. It is an amazing exercise to develop your shoulders and triceps.

Muscles Worked

Shoulder and Triceps

How

-Sit on a bench with your back rested.

-Lift the dumbbells next to your shoulders with the palms facing forward.

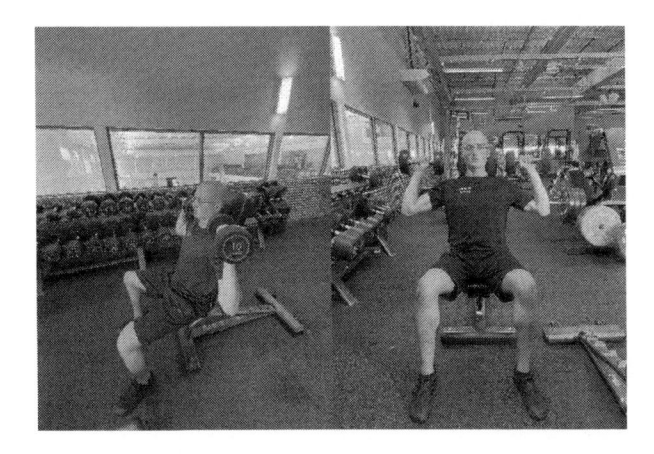

-Push the dumbbells over your head, finishing with arms straight.

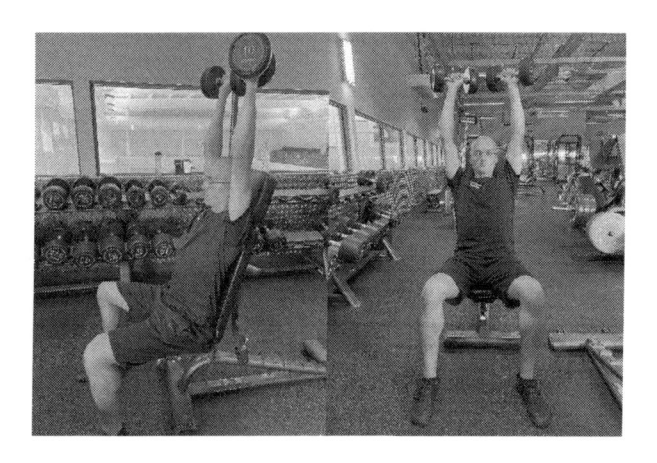

-Lower down slowly into starting position and go again.

Regression/Progression

You can start as low as 2.5kg for each dumbbell and once you get to 8/10 clean repetitions, I suggest you increase the load.

Common Mistakes to Avoid

-Not closing the dumbbell together on top of the movement but keep them over your shoulders or wider (they should be over your head).

-Pushing them in front of you/diagonally rather than over your head.

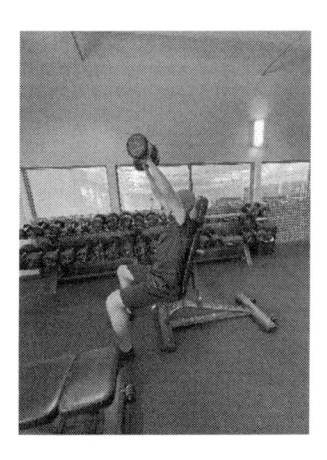

Alternatives

-Shoulder Press (page 30)

-Dips (page 121)

How would it feel?

You will feel it more on the anterior part of your shoulders when you push from the bottom, while at the top you will feel it more on your triceps, especially close to your elbow joint.

DB Arnold Press

Why

The Arnold Press is a fantastic movement to develop strong and big shoulders. You will work your shoulders through a bigger range of motion that you would in a common overhead press. The rotation during the movement transfers the weight from the anterior head to the lateral head, making this exercise an excellent choice.

Muscles Worked

Shoulder and Triceps

How

-Sit with your back laying on the bench and grab two dumbbells.

-Start with dumbbells just in front of your shoulders with palms facing you.

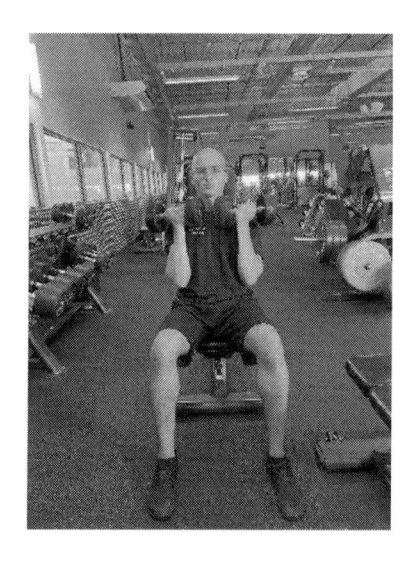

-Push the dumbbells up, and while you do that rotate it.

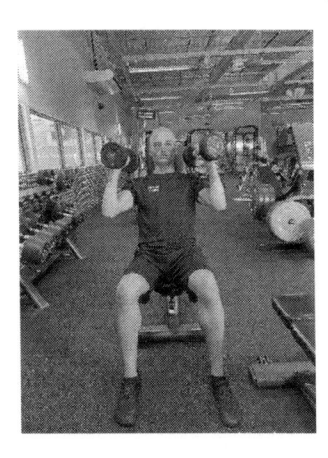

-Finish the movement with the palms facing in front of you and arms straight.

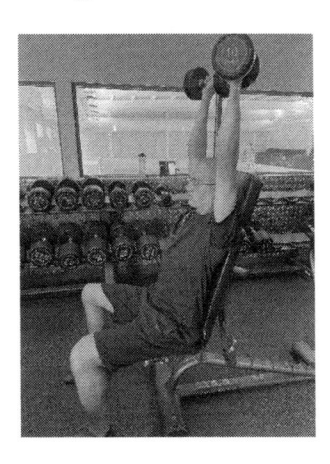

Regression/Progression

- Simply increase or decrease the weight. Some people go heavy in this one (6reps) while others prefer staying between 10-12 reps. I personally would suggest starting light with high reps, and then, once you master the movement you can perform it at low reps.

-Moreover, you might decide to do the standing variation that require more core strength and body awareness. In this case make sure to squeeze your glutes and abdominal muscles to keep your trunk straight. By doing this you will probably be able to lift less weight. However, the exercise will be more effective in working your core as well as protecting your low back.

Common Mistakes to Avoid

- Not rotating properly. To make this exercise effective you must rotate as you are coming up rather than rotate at the bottom or at the top of the movement.

- Losing tension. Do not bring the elbows too low at the bottom as you would lose tension on your shoulders and put it on your biceps (it is not what you want with this exercise)

-Doing it too heavy. Put aside your ego and focus on technique first!

-Push the dumbbells in front of you rather than over your head. This will put more pressure on your anterior delts as well as shoulder and elbow joins and reducing the work of your traps and triceps.

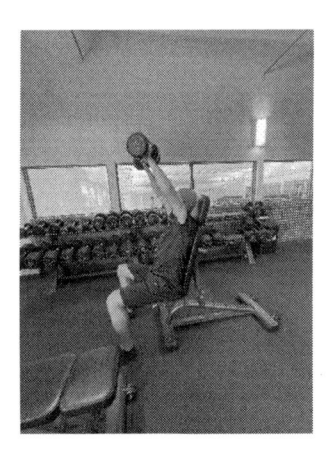

Alternatives

-DB Overhead Press (page 74)

-Shoulder Press (page 30)

-Pike Pushups (page 124)

How would it feel?

You should feel it like the overhead press but with more emphasis on the lateral part of the shoulder. I like to think at this exercise like a calf raise of the upper body. Once the dumbbells are over your head squeeze voluntarily your shoulders and then come back into starting position.

PULL EXERCISES

DB Row

Why
It is a basic horizontal pull that works your back muscles as well as your anterior delts and biceps. Unlike resistance machine, you need stabilisation to do it, requiring other muscle on your core to work to keep you balanced.

Muscles Worked

Back, Biceps and posterior part of the shoulder (last two muscles to a much lesser degree)

How

(Let's do it on our left side)

-Put your right knee and your right arm on a bench (or other support).

-Keep your back straight and almost parallel on the floor.

-Pick a dumbbell with the other hand.

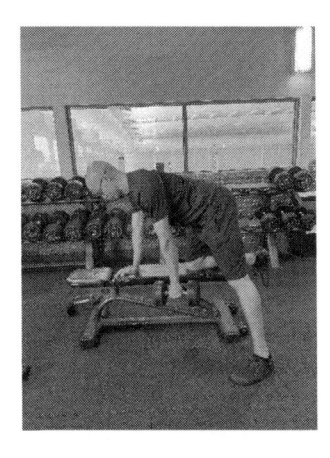

-Lift the dumbbell towards your trunk by keeping your back straight and chest out.

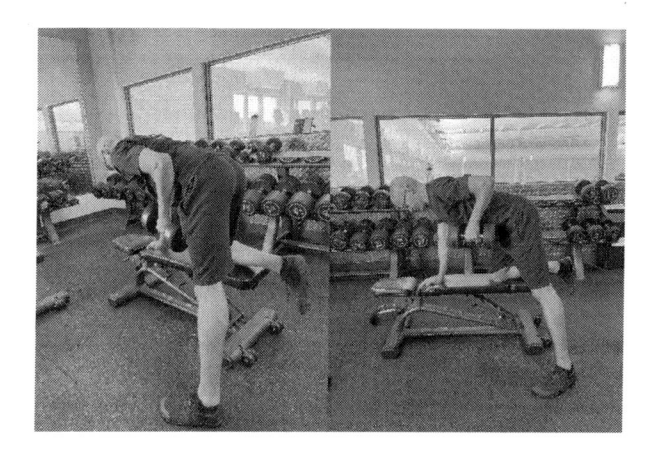

-hold it one second on top squeezing your back muscles.

-Go back into starting position slowly, and repeat.

Regression/Progression

It is a simple movement that does not require progression or regression. In fact, the only variable you can change is the load. (Yes, you might also change the tempo of the exercise, but it would not be necessary and would complicate your workout).

Common Mistakes to Avoid

-Keep your back rounded instead of having back straight.

-Lifting the dumbbell up towards your shoulder (ideally you want to think to bring the dumbbell towards the pocket, like in the image above).

Alternatives

-Seated Row (page 41)

-Inverted Row (page 129)

How would it feel?

It might be that for the first few times you do not really feel your back working a lot. A quick tip would be to imagine squeezing your back muscle every time you pull. In fact, imagine your shoulder blades touching each other while keeping your chest out. I will guarantee you that the effect will be immediate!

BB Row

Why

Barbell Row is one of the greatest exercises to develop a thick and strong back. It is a compound movement that will also enhance the strength on your biceps, traps an all the muscle around your trunk. It is easy to overload and by improving in this exercise you can be sure to develop a strong and aesthetic back.

Muscles Worked

Back, and also posterior part of the shoulder and biceps (last two muscles to a much lesser degree)

How

-Grab the barbell from the rack (the height should roughly about knee level) with your hands slightly wider than shoulder width apart with an overhand grip (palms facing the floor, not you).

If you do not use a rack, but you lift it from the floor, make sure that the bar is above your mid foot.

You can also do it with palms facing you and hands shoulder width apart to work more your biceps rather than upper back.

-Pull the bar up to start the exercise while keeping it very close to your body (the farther forward the more stress you will put on your low back).

-Slightly bend your knees and lean forward/ push your butt back by keeping your back straight and chest out (DO NOT hunch).

How forward? For a max back activation and development overtime you would stay almost horizontal to the ground. However, most of the people do not have the mobility on their hip/hamstring region, and strength in their spine to get into this position safely. As a rule: Lean forward as much as you comfortably can while keeping a neutral spine (you naturally have a slight arch on your low back).

-Start with your arms straight.

All teaching points above are summarized in this photo below.

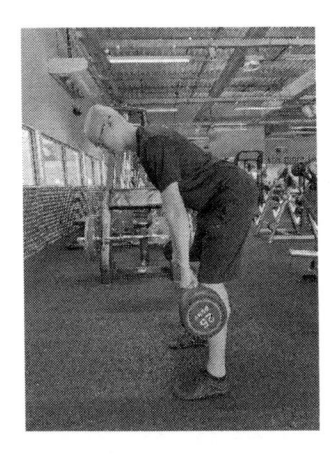

-Pull the barbell towards the area between your belly button and top of your abs.

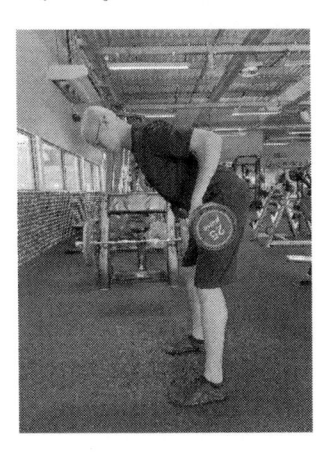

Note: for simplicity, I would say the belly button is a good idea where to pull. However, for maximal efficacy, pull the barbell with a position that let your elbows go behind your body as much as you can, while keeping your elbows tucked to your body.

- Squeeze on top for a second (focus on squeezing your back muscle and shoulder blades touching each other as you do so).

- Go back down slowly into starting position and repeat it for the desired reps.

Regression/Progression

-Simply increase or decrease the reps. Anywhere between 6 and 12 reps works well. This is the type of exercise that it is better to perform at relatively low reps (6-8 reps). It does not mean you have to perform it heavy all the time, but to maximise its benefits some heavy rows are necessary.

Common Mistakes to Avoid

-Round your upper back. By doing that you can injure yourself as well as not getting the benefits of the exercise. In fact, by keeping your back straight and your chest out, you will be able to squeeze your back once you pull the bar towards you.

Another reason because you might round your back is because you are leaning too much forward. It happens mainly because the hamstrings are too tight and so you must round your low back to get into position. How to solve it? Simply lean forward less (and work on your hamstring strength/mobility with exercise such as Nordic Curl, page 159, and RDL, Page 168)

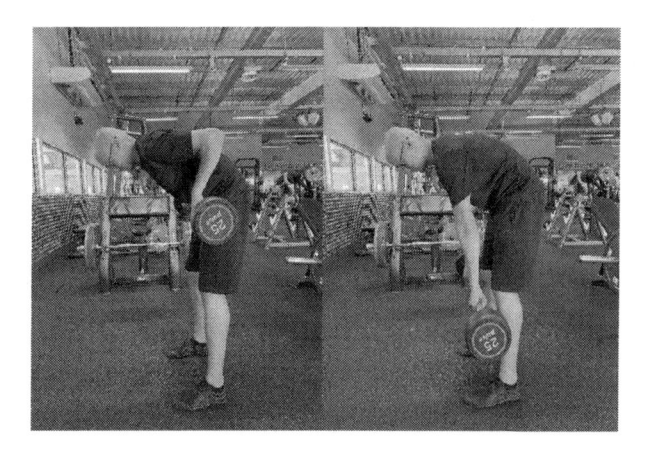

-Staying too upright with your trunk. If you do so, there will be less lats engagement, resulting into more an upper back /traps exercise (which is not wrong, but it is not the main point of this exercise).

-Flaring out the elbow too much. If you do flare out you might lose tension on your lats, which is one of the main muscles involved in the exercise. Keep your elbows tucked while doing the exercise.

- Starting the movement from the biceps. It is not only less efficient than pulling from your back but also might lead to tendon injury when the load is heavy. So, how do you avoid this? At the starting position, once you un-rack the barbell, and you still have your arms straight, contract your triceps before to pull the barbell. By doing this, you will activate your lats from the very start.

Alternatives

-DB Row (page 83)

-Seated Row (page 41)

-Inverted Rows (page 129)

How would it feel?

To feel this exercise maximally try not only to pull the bar towards you but imagine that you would break the bar and turn it externally. This way you will easily engage your lats to a bigger extent. Moreover, like many other exercises that requires pushing and pulling using a dumbbell/barbell, squeezing the bar as hard as you can, will enhance your nervous system and strength.

Note: if you are a beginner inn this exercise you might find this cue overwhelming. I that so, forget about it for a few weeks, and try to incorporate it again later.

DB Pullover

Why

Dumbbell Pullover is not only a great exercise for your lats, but also helps with your posture. In fact, this exercise will stretch your lats and allow you to get actively into range of motion that you have not probably explored in a long time. Moreover, having a wide back is something that most guys want, and this exercise really target the lats and teres major (that little muscle on top of the lats) that work on your V-shape.

Muscles Worked

Back

How

-Upper back on a bench and grab the dumbbell holding it by the inside of one extremity just over your chest.

-Bench just resting below the middle of the head (so you do not create any stress on your neck).

-Hips up levelled with your body.

-Shoulders rolled back at starting position.

-Let the weight go down and you will feel a nice stretch on your lats.

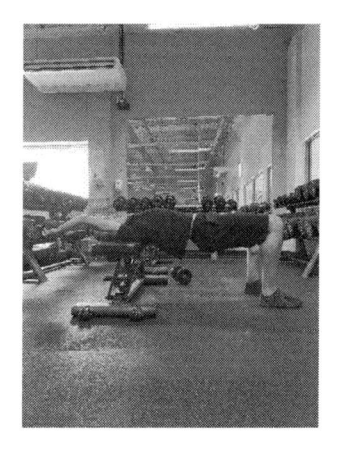

-From bottom position you are going to drive your palms onto the air up (away from your body, keeping arm straight).

- Stop with your weight over your chin and go again. You might extend the range of motion a bit more and that would not be wrong. Be aware that in that way you will engage your upper chest and lose some tension on your back (not a terrible thing if this is what you want).

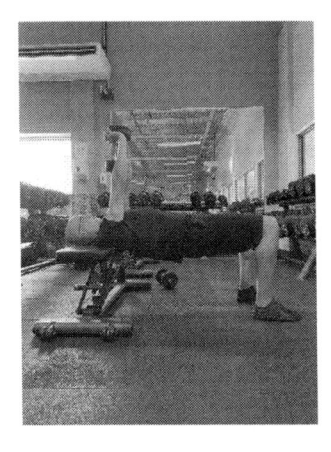

Regression/Progression

Simply adjust the load to make it easier or more difficult.

Common Mistakes to Avoid

-Do not dip the hips too low.

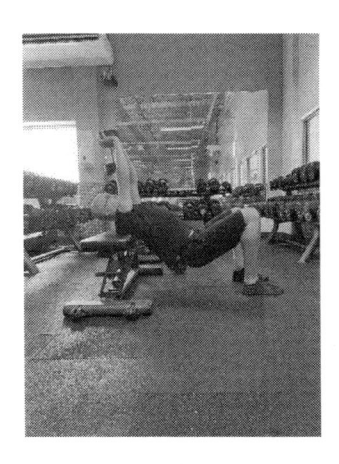

-Do not have your shoulders push forward. It would put unnecessary stress on your shoulder joint and would be less effective for your back.

- Do not grab the dumbbell as you normal would when doing other exercise. By doing that you will work more on your grip, and you probably end up doing less reps as your forearm will not allow you to complete your sets.

-Bend your arms when pulling the weight up. This would result in ore triceps activation rather than lats activation.

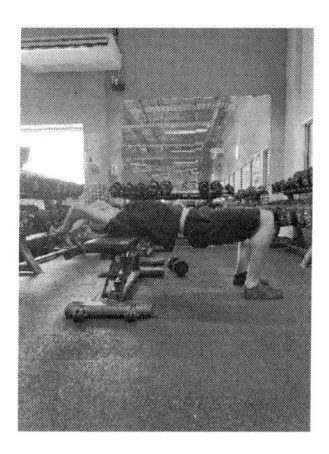

Alternatives

-Lat Pull down (page 44)

-Chin-ups (page 126)

How would it feel?

You will feel a nice stretch on your lats, outside part of your back. It will be a new feeling, and I bet you will like the sensation after having performed a few sets of this. Many people when they first perform this exercise notice straightaway how it helps with their posture
(Especially who tend to slouch will notice incredible benefits).

CORE EXERCISES

Plank Dumbbell Drag

Why

This exercise will not only work your core like a normal Plank would do, but also you will have to fight not to rotate your body. I would suggest you build up to at least 60" Plank before doing this.

Muscles Worked
Core muscles (Rectus Abdominis aka six-pack and Obliques mainly)

How
-Start in a plank position with arms straight with a dumbbell next to one of your sides.

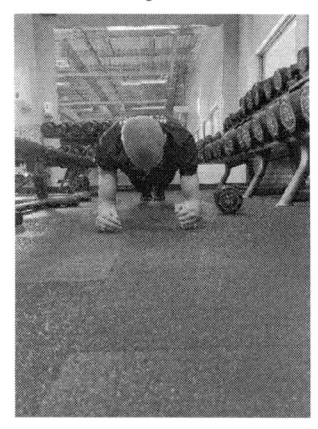

-With the opposite hand pick the dumbbell and move it to the other side.

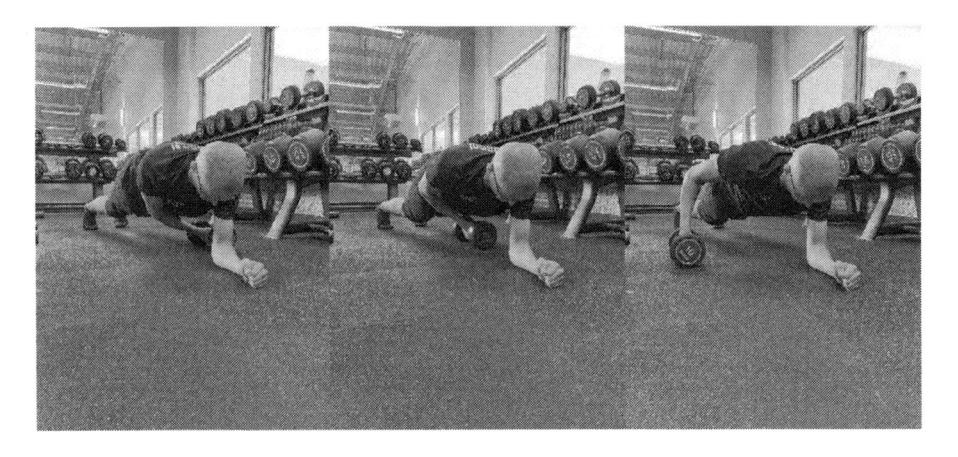

-Come back into starting position by having your arms straight below your shoulders.

-Do it again on the opposite side.

Regression/Progression

In this exercise there are not big regression or progression. Once you can move a dumbbell of 5/10 kg side to side for 10 times, you are mastering this movement and it is probably time to doing some other exercises.

Common Mistakes to Avoid

-Performing the reps fast. Ding it fast and accumulate more reps/ finish the reps in less time is not beneficial. When performing core exercises is important the balance and coordination aspect. Doing it slow and controlled. Your goal should be to master the movement.

-Moving the hips. When moving the dumbbell is important that your hips are still facing the floor, otherwise the benefits of this exercise will not be present.

How would it feel?

You will feel it slightly more challenging than a plank as it requires more body control and awareness.

Renegade Row

Why

It is an amazing exercise to develop a strong core and control. It works your core in an anti-extension position as well as anti-rotation. Being able to resist to rotational forces is important for many athletes (or people that want to train like one). For regular gymgoers this can be a good exercise to work your core in a different way than the normal plank, side plank, Russian twist that you have probably been doing for ages…(Instead, if you are just starting working out now I would suggest you to stick to Plank and Side plank (page xx) until you get a strong foundation of at least 30" each before approaching this exercise).

Muscles Worked

Core Muscles

How

-Start in a pushup position (arms below shoulders, feet close, body in a straight-line position) with one hand holding dumbbell.

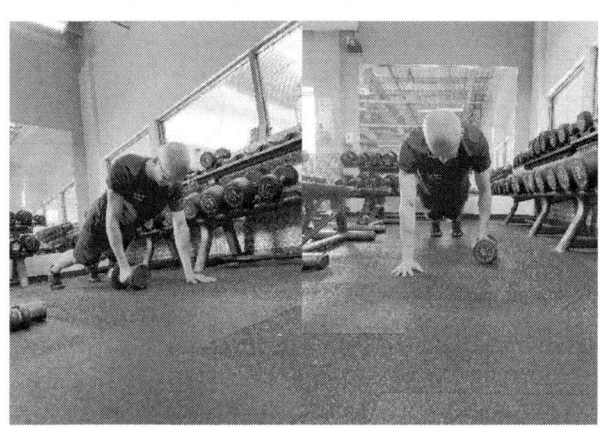

-Pull one dumbbell to the side of the hip.

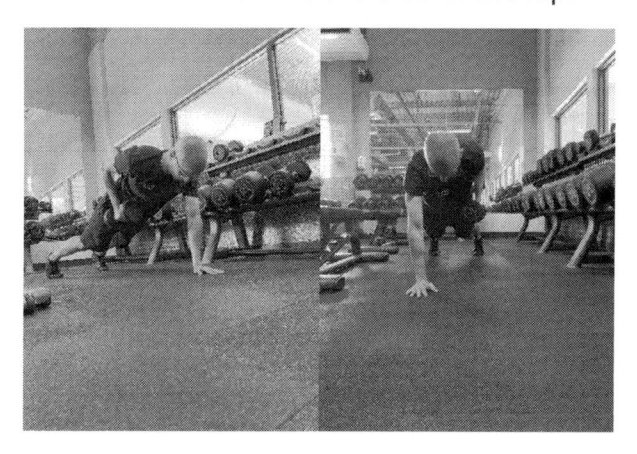

-Come back into starting position and repeat (make sure to work on the other side too!).

Regression/Progression

-Wider stance will make the exercise easier. The closer your feet the more difficult.

Common Mistakes to Avoid

-Opening the hips. The hips ideally should always face the ground. That way you will engage your abs more.

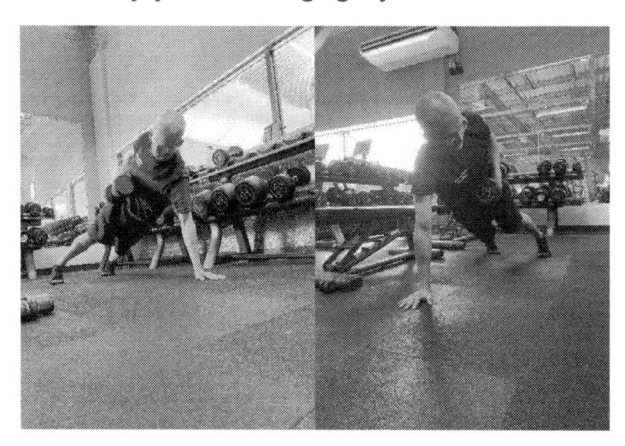

How would it feel?

When performing this movement, you really have to focus on having a stable and fixed position on hips and shoulders without any rotation. That's key to maximise the efficacy of this exercise.

ARMS EXERCISES

Bicep Curl

Why

Great accessory workout to work on your biceps. It is 1/3 of your arms and train it especially will mainly help for aesthetics and grip strength (in case you practice some sports that requires it).

Muscles Worked

Biceps

How

You can do standing or seated, with Dumbbells or Barbell. I personally would recommend you the standing version with dumbbells. This is because you can explore more range of motion without any discomfort that a barbell or the seated version might cause.

-Grab the dumbbells with the palms facing away from you.

-From the starting position, lift your forearms while keeping your elbow tucked to the side.

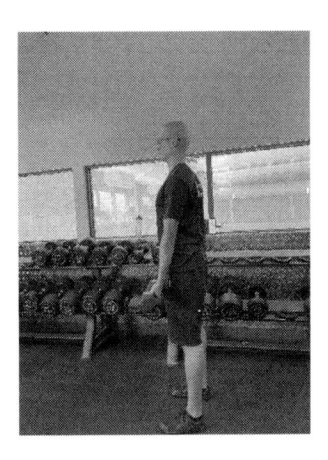

-Once your wrist is very close to your shoulder, squeeze it on top.

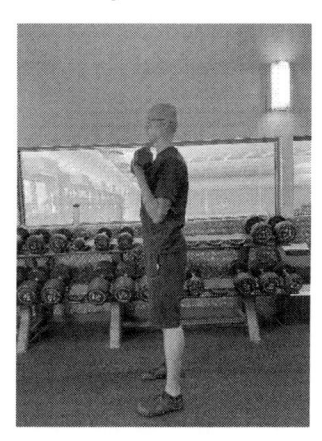

-Then go back into starting position.

Regression/Progression

-You can simply use a lighter load and perform the exercise that way. Once you can do 10+ reps easily, it is time to increase load.

Common Mistakes to Avoid

-Moving the elbows forward. By doing this, you will be able to lift more weight or doing more reps as the shoulder will assist the movement. However, it will be less effective, so I would not suggest you do it.

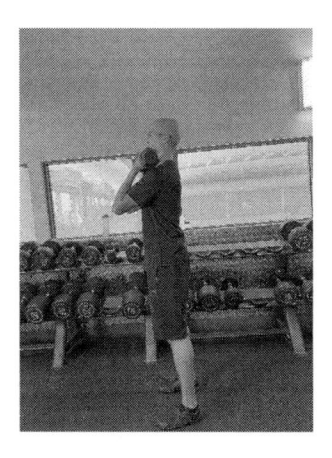

-Not locking out the rep on top. You have to lock out every rep and squeeze your bicep for 1-2 ". That way you will enhance your bicep strength and hypertrophy.

-Bouncing back from the bottom position. If you use momentum the rep will be easier. Ideally, you should do it slowly and controlled to avoid injury and maximise your results long term.

-Leaning backwards. This might cause low back pain. If you do this it might be that you are using too much weight (or that you are doing too many reps and your bicep is not that strong yet, so other muscles have to compensate).

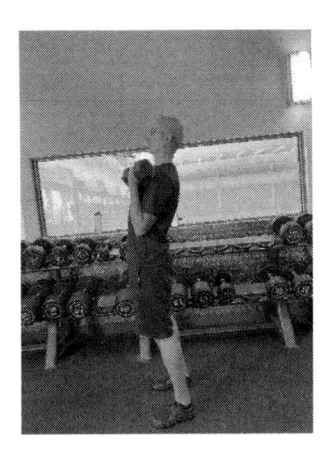

How would it feel?

The feeling, regardless of your training expertise would be a contraction on your biceps. You might also feel some tension on your forearms when lifting the weight up.

Dumbbell Skull crusher

Why

It is an effective exercise to really isolate the triceps. It is good for any levels, whether you are an advanced lifters and you want to step up your hypertrophy in your arms, or you just started and you want to utilize this exercise to help you get stronger, and eventually perform your first pushups!

You can also do it with a barbell or any barbell variations. Personally, I will suggest you start with dumbbells because you will have a neutral grip and you do not need to rotate your wrist. So, no wrist mobility (and shoulders to some extent) is needed, therefore applicable for everyone). Also, you can do it double arms at the same time. To start with, I would do it single arm so you can assist yourself with the other hand, getting the mechanics of the movement well.

Muscles Worked

Triceps

How

-Lay down on a bench and grab the dumbbells with a neutral grip (It simply means that as you lay down your palms is facing in, like in photo).

Ideally you would also grab the dumbbells towards the bottom (like showed in picture) so when you flip it, the weight will be resting on your hands, releasing some pressure from your wrist.

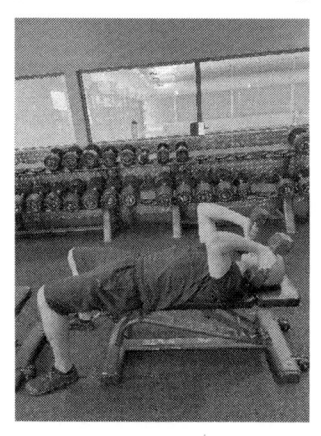

-Start with your elbows in a straight position.

-Keep your elbows in a fixed position while doing the movement. It must stay vertical to the ground (other variations might have the elbow in different positions, but for now keep it vertical).

-Lower Down the weight slowly down. Try to go down in four seconds. At the bottom should be right by your ear (or at least with your forearm bent at 90°). Then, push back up and extend your elbow.

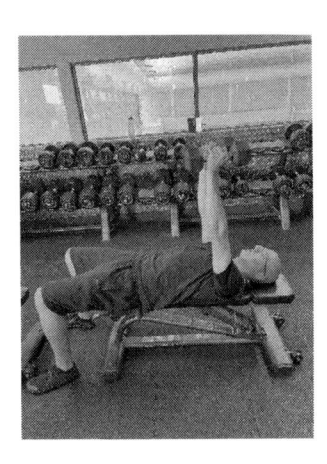

-Once you extend your elbows keep the triceps flexed. Otherwise, all the pressure will go on your joints.

Regression/Progression

-Simply increase or decrease the load. Once you cand o more than 10 reps with a given weight, I would increase the load with a heavier dumbbell.

Common Mistakes to Avoid

-Do not move back and forth shoulder and elbow while performing the movement. It will engage other muscle that are not required when performing this accessory exercise. If you struggle to keep your elbows in a fixed position, you can use the non-working hand to stabilize the elbow.

How would it feel?

You will feel a nice stretch at the back of your arms as you resist on the way down. Then as you push back up it will be challenging in the middle part of the range. Some people might experience some discomfort on your elbows. If your technique is right, it might be because you are using too much weight.

If that is the case pick up a lighter weight and perform more reps (this will give more blood flow to the muscle and connective tissue).

SPECIAL OFFER: do you feel like you need an extra help and accountability for your fitness journey? Go to **avfitness99.wixsite.com** or DM me on **Instagram- avfitness99-** and see the different possibilities that you can get from Online Coaching.

PERSONALISED PLAN

Tailored 4 weeks plan based on your goals and gym frequency

--Free Zoom Consultation

-4 weeks plan

-Video Tutorial for Each Exercise

MONTHLY COACHING
Perfect for people serious to get fit

-Free Zoom Consultation

-4 weeks plan

-Video Tutorial for Each Exercise

-Nutritional Guidelines

-Training Check 2x/weekly

-Answer to any question within 24 hours

ELITE COACHING
Full accountability for training / lifestyle

-Free Zoom Consultation

-4 weeks personalised plan

-Video Tutorial for each exercise

-Nutritional advice

-Lifestyle advice

-Daily text for workout

-Daily text for diet/lifestyle

-24/7 Support and accountability

-2 Zoom individualized HIIT Workout a month

Now let's go back to the book!

*The offer might change overtime. Look at my Instagram or website to stay in touch **with the most recent updates.**

AVFITNESS99

SCAN ME

LOWER BODY EXERCISES

-BB Squat

Why

It is considered the king of the exercise. Squats work everything (lower body wise). Also, it engages your core as a stabilizer. It translates very well into sprinting and jumping.

The stronger you are squatting, the less likely you will have knee pain (if you do it with the right technique as I am going to show you), the faster you'll be, the stronger your legs will be, and the easier you'll perform any type of exercise and daily life activities.

There is no reason you should not be squatting!

Muscles Worked

Quads, Glutes (and many other muscles playing a minor role such as calves, hamstrings, core, upper back and lats)

How

-Before un-racking the weight, make sure it is roughly shoulder-height. You should be your knees to get into position, otherwise you adjust the bar too high on the squat rack (which is also going to be uncomfortable when you put the barbell back on it).

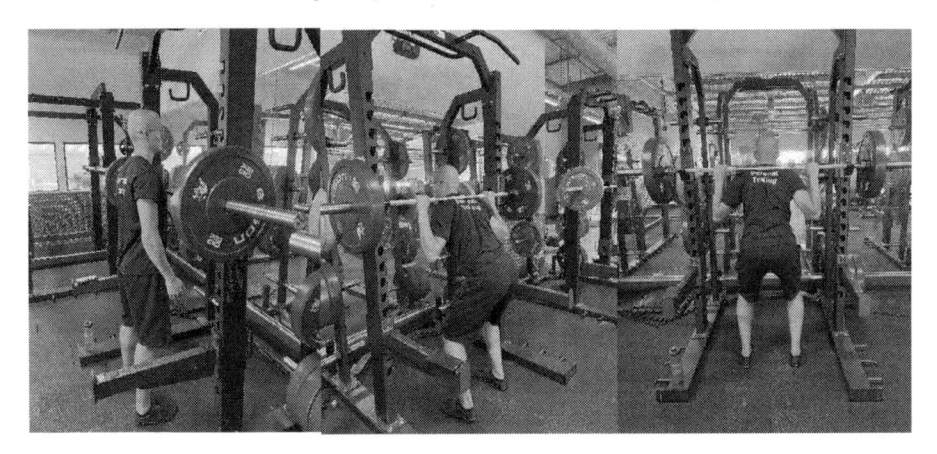

-Put your feet hip width apart with toes pointing slightly forward. Grab the bar slightly wider than shoulder width apart.

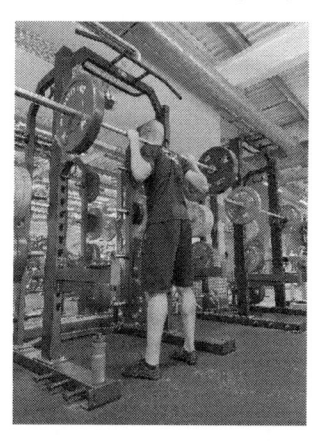

-Once you squat focus on three contact points of your feet on the ground: Heel, below the big toe and just below the pinkie. These three points apply pressure on the ground (it will help you to stabilize)

-Squat down (at least 90°) slowly and controlled, pause for a moment at the bottom, and then push back up.

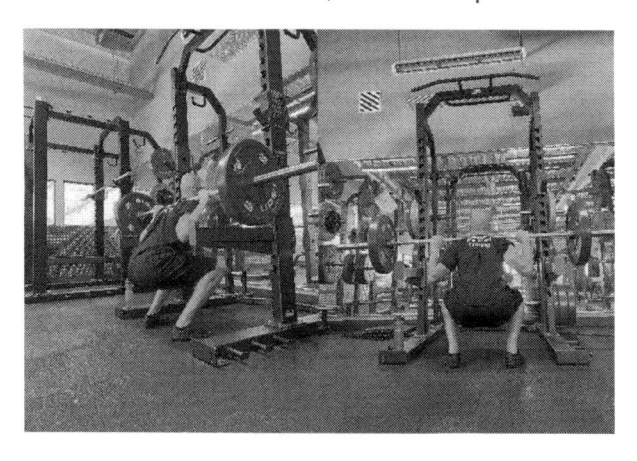

Regression/Progression

1)Bodyweight

2)Holding a Dumbbell/Kettlebell close to your chest 3)

Barbell

Once you get to the barbell version with good technique the progression would be mainly increasing load and repetitions overtime.

Alternatives

You can do:

-Bulgarian Split Squat (page 138)

-Lunges (go to page 113)

-Front Squat (Holding the bar in front of you rather than on your back. It requires more core strength as well as recruiting more quads)

Common Mistakes to Avoid

-Do not go too low (drop the weight and squat appropriately.9

-Leaning forward too much (it is usually due to lack of ankle mobility. You can fix it by improving in the ATG Split Squat and ankle mobility exercises. Look at pages 148 and 162 to learn more

-Bringing the bar forward (this is usually a problem related to ankle and hip mobility. For ankle mobility look at the ATG Split Squat as mentioned before, while for the hip mobility look at "Hip exercises" at page 165). Ideally the bar should be above your mid foot the entire time of the execution.

Alternatives

-Leg Press (page 54)

-DB Lunges (page 113)

-Box Pistol Squat (page 136)

-Bulgarian Split Squat (page 138)

How would it feel?

Whilst doing it, you must be focus on:

-the contact points of your feet on the ground.

-Keeping the bar above your midfoot, so it is centered.

-Go low enough (at least 90°angle, with hips in line with your knees)

BB Hip Thrust

Why

Hip thrust is a fantastic exercise to develop strong and powerful glutes.

Moreover, it is simple to lean the technique, it is a very safe exercise, and it can be overload quite quickly!

Muscles Worked

Glutes

How

-Bar on your pelvis, ready to initiate the movement.

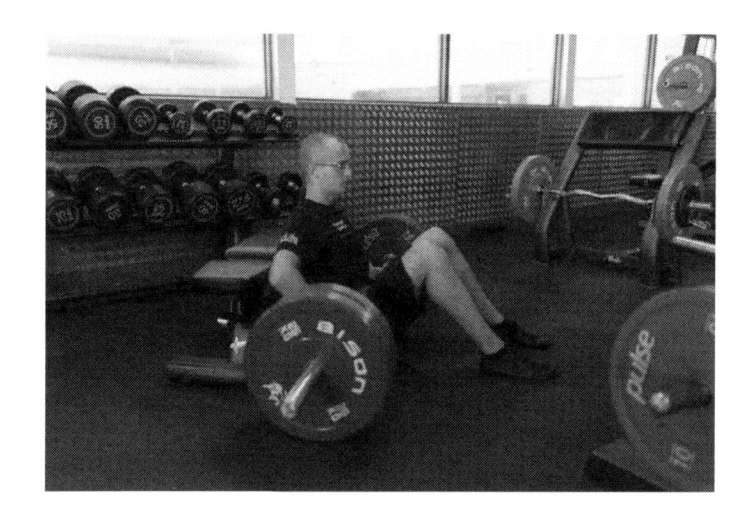

-Put your upper back against the box and shins vertical to the ground.

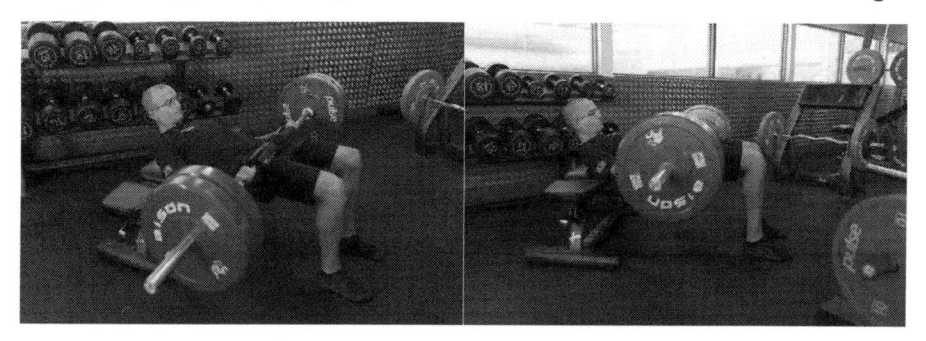

-REMEMBER: Squeeze your glutes at the top of the movement. This is key to maximise their growth and activation.

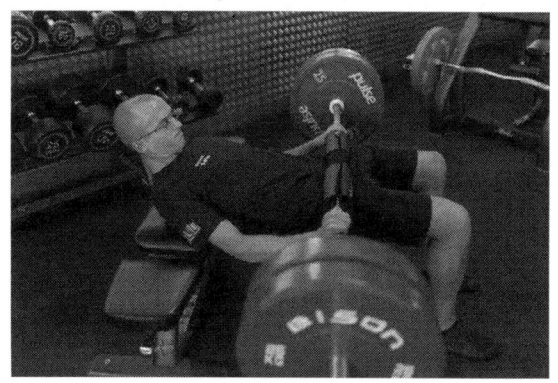

-Go down slowly.

(Stop going down once you have to bend other joints other than your hips, like knees or extend your back)

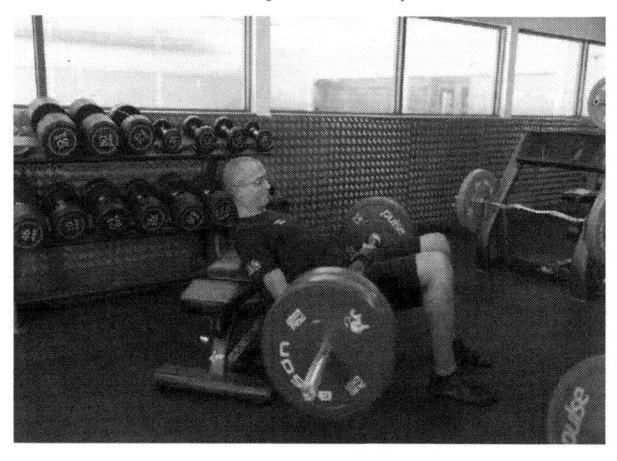

Regression/Progression

-You will probably want to start with the sandbag (10/15kg)

-Then you will start using a barbell and overload it.

Common Mistakes

-Not locking out on top of the movement

-Having your feet too far or too close from the box. Shins must stay vertical to the ground

Alternatives

-BB RDL (page 110)

How would it feel?

You should feel most of the work on your glutes. If you do not: Try squeeze for a couple of second on top, focusing on pushing through your heels, drive your knees out when you do it...Just one of those three tips would be enough to have your glutes on fire!

BB RDL

Why

RDL, or Romanian Deadlift, is one of the best exercises for the posterior chain (mainly hamstring and glutes, but also your back will work).

It allows to work your hamstrings by extending the hip and working your glutes in a stretched position (unlike hip thrust, for example).

I would like to think about this exercise as a loaded stretch. In fact, the connective tissue is lengthened as you go down. From that position, where we are at our weakest, we must be able to exert strength. It is a fantastic exercise to bulletproof your hamstrings as well as getting stronger.

It has tons a carryover on exercises such as back extension, hip thrust, deadlift, sumo deadlift and even pullups.

Muscles Worked

Hamstrings and Glutes

How

-Keep your back straight.

-Grab the bar slightly wider than shoulder width (your grip should be just outside your knees).

-Knee slightly bent in a fixed position throughout the entire movement.

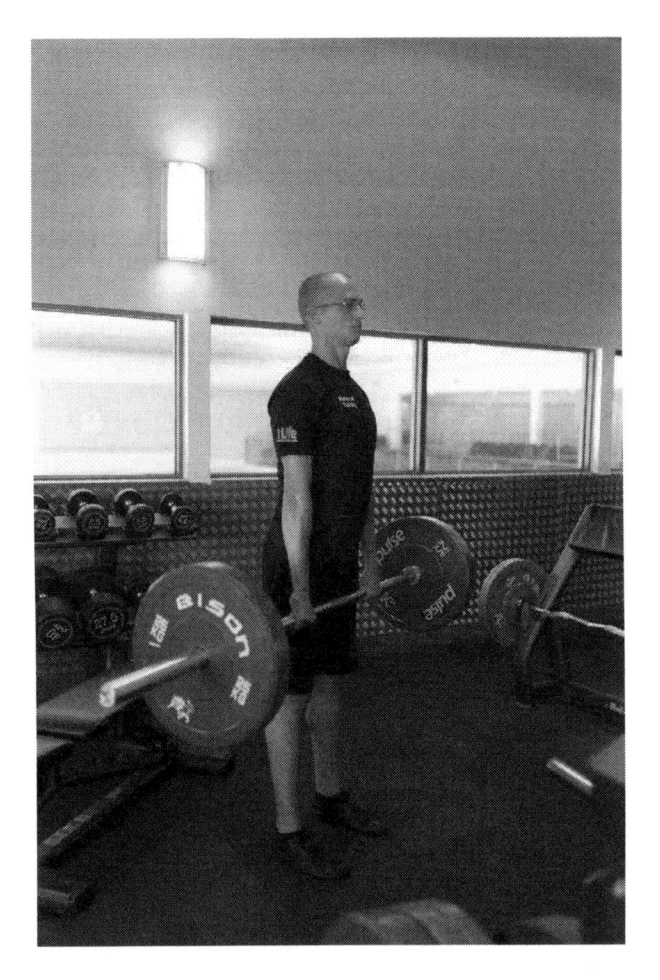

-Push the glutes back on the way down feeling a stretch on your hamstrings.

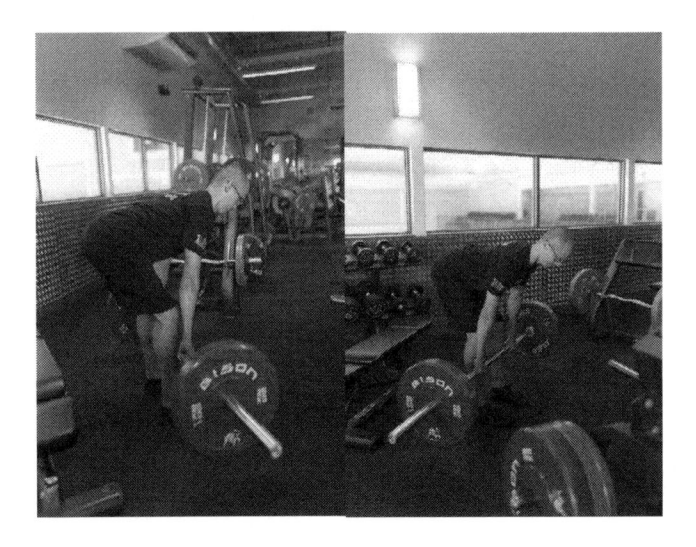

-Push back up hinging at the hips, pushing your feet (especially the heel) against the floor.

-Keep the bar close to your body throughout the entire movement

Regression/Progression

You can start with dumbbells, and then progress into a barbell.
A variation that you can do is to do it unilateral (requires more balance/coordination but give less possibility to overload).
A progression that you can try is to elevate your feet as to increase the range of motion.

Common Mistakes

-Rounding your back (Rounding your spine is not wrong.... in fact, exercises such as Jefferson Curls are great to do. However, during RDL your back should be straight)

Alternatives

Glute Bridge (page xx) You might also do Leg Curl (page xx) or Nordic Curl (page xx). However, these two exercises do not work your glutes but only the hamstrings, unlike RDL and Glute Bridge.

How would it feel?

-As you go down, you will feel a nice stretch on your posterior chain. Once you push the barbell back up, you will feel the glutes helping to close the movement. You might also feel it on your back and grip.
If you do not feel it on your glutes when you push the bar up (but only in your hamstrings), once you push the bar back up, focus on pushing with your heels on the floor rather than your entire foot. This should do the magic!

Instead, if you feel it on your low back, chances are that you are going to low according to your mobility and strength. For most people going just below the kneecap it more than enough to get results.
It is an intense exercise, so plan it into your training accordingly.

DB Lunges

Why

Lunges, just like Squats, is an exercise that target different leg muscles at the same time, as well as engaging your core to stabilise yourself during the movement.

Muscles Worked

Glutes and Quads.

How

You can perform it in different ways. I am going to show you how to perform Walking Lunges.

-Start with two dumbbells on your hands.

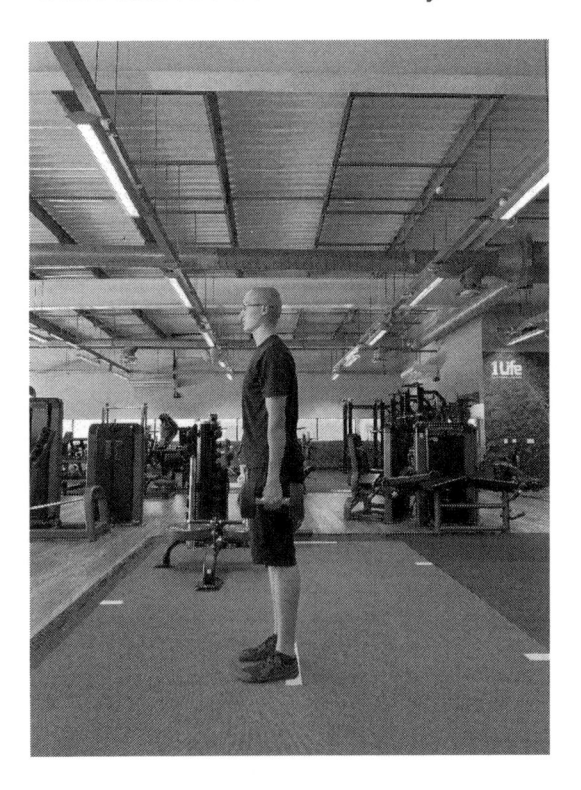

-Step forward with one leg so to create 90° at the knee and ankle of both legs.

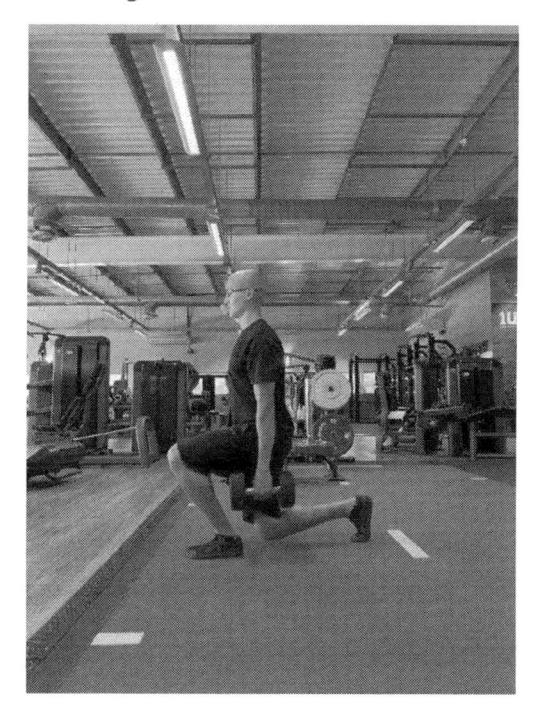

-Push with the leg in front to stand up again.

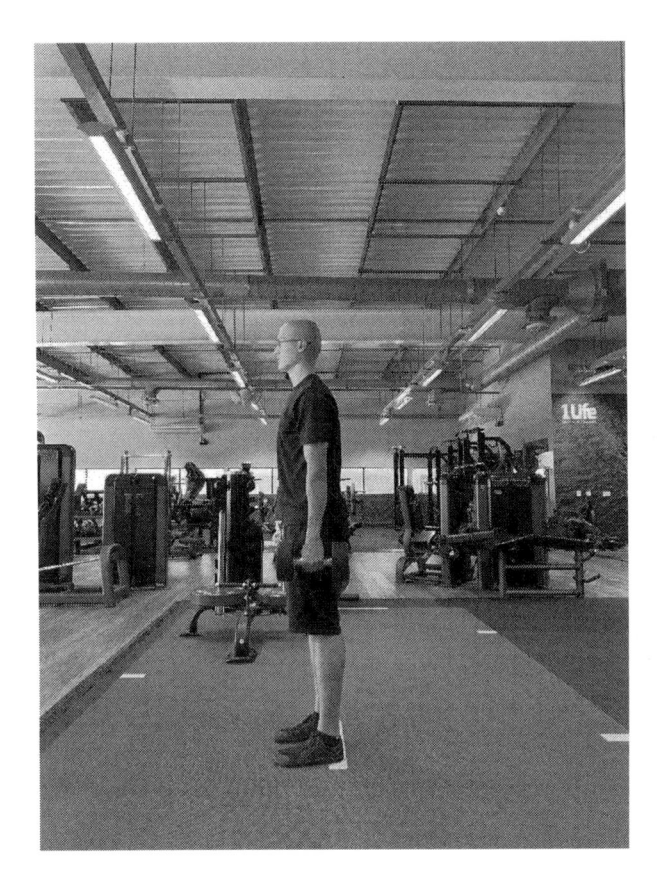

-Reset and go again.

Regression/Progression

Start by doing this exercise bodyweight. Then you can use two dumbbells to hold on the side (keeping arm straight). Eventually you will use a barbell on your back.

Common Mistakes to Avoid

-Not going low enough.

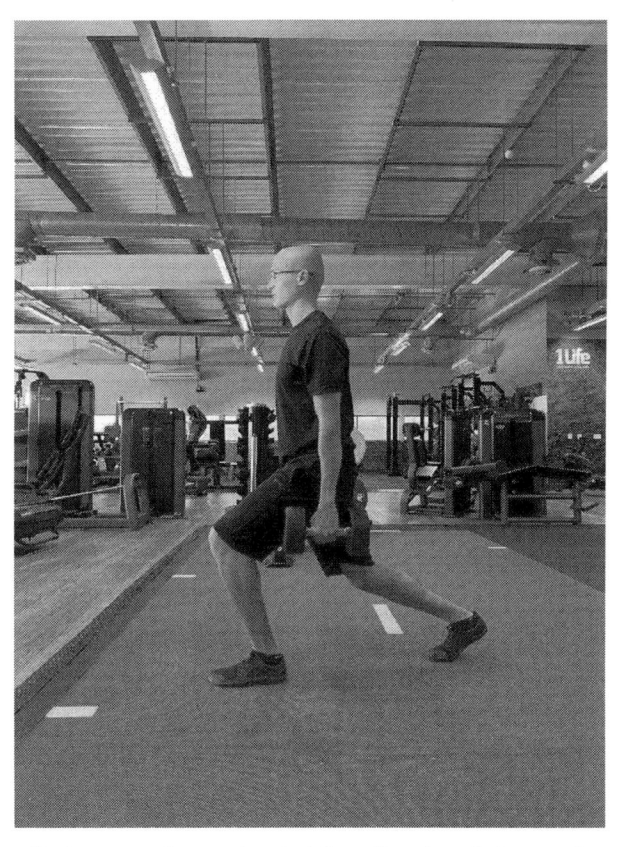

-Going too low aka letting the back knee touch the floor.

-Having an arm on your front thigh as you push back up (arms must be on the side).

Alternatives

-Leg Press (page 54)

-BB Squat (page 103)

-Box Pistol Squat (page 136)

How Would it Feel?

You will feel it a lot on your front leg as you do it. Not only the quads will work but also your glutes. Moreover, you can play around with this exercise by changing the position of your trunk. If you lean forward slightly when performing the movement you will feel it more on your glutes, while keeping your trunk upright will benefit more your thighs.

BODYWEIGHT EXERCISES

Here we are! Bodyweight exercises are probably the foundation of exercise. Not only you will not need expensive equipment to do them, but they not only work on your strength but also on your mobility, coordination, and balance. I would say that every single person should be doing some sort of bodyweight exercise.

In fact, an old person can benefit from them to get stronger based on his/her bodyweight to make sure he/she is still fit to move, walk, do stairs daily. For a regular gym goer also, it is important to be aware of their body, and bodyweight provide this benefit (unfortunately, you see many people being able to lift crazy number of weights in some exercises, and then struggling doing a single pull up).

UPPER BODY PUSH EXERCISES

Push-ups

Why

It is a basic exercise that allows you to get stronger relative to your bodyweight. The entry barrier for this exercise is very low and everyone can do it (or at least a regression of it). Moreover, it will improve your cardiovascular system as many studies showed. Being strong in the pushups will have great results not only in terms of upper body and core strength but also for your heart's health.

Muscles Worked

Chest, Triceps, Shoulder (anterior part) and Core

How

-Go into a plank position with arms straight

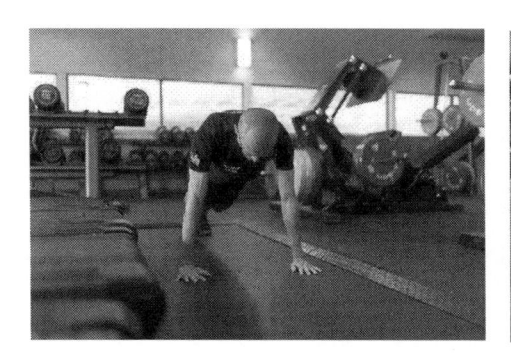

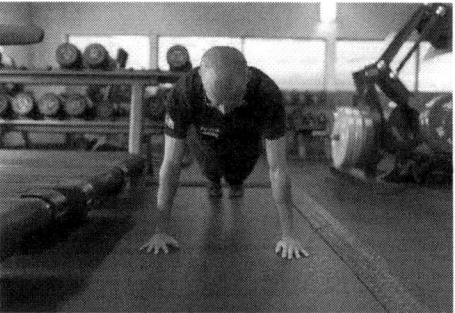

Put your wrist/hands just below your shoulder, and from there, put them a bit wider.

-Lower down by keeping your core straight.

-Bring your chest in between your arms (Do not flare out the elbows too much).

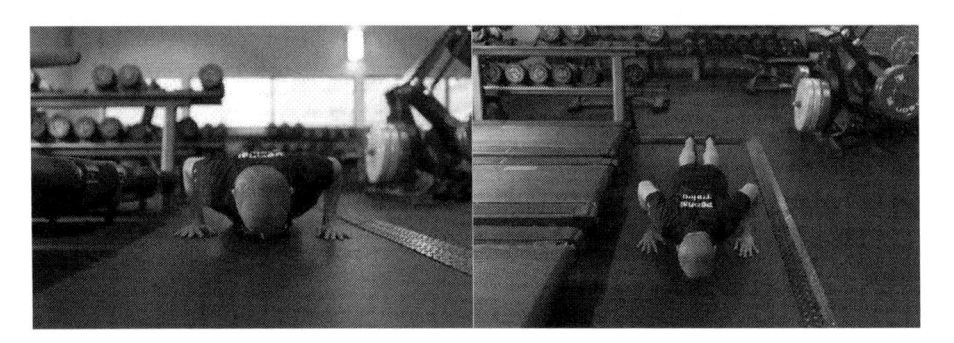

-Pause half a second at the bottom, and then push back up.

Regression/Progression

Knee Push-ups are used by many people, but they do not have a great carryover on pushups (the lever is different and even though you might get to do 10/15 knee pushups, I think you would be still struggling getting to one good pushups).

-Elevating the hand positioning is the best way to go.

-Overtime you can decrease the height until you do it on the floor.

As a progression, once you can do 15+ pushups easy, you can:

-Elevate your feet on a box

-Try diamond Pushups

-Put weight on your back (with a partner)

-Use dumbbells to increase range of motion

Common Mistakes to Avoid

-Flare out the elbows.

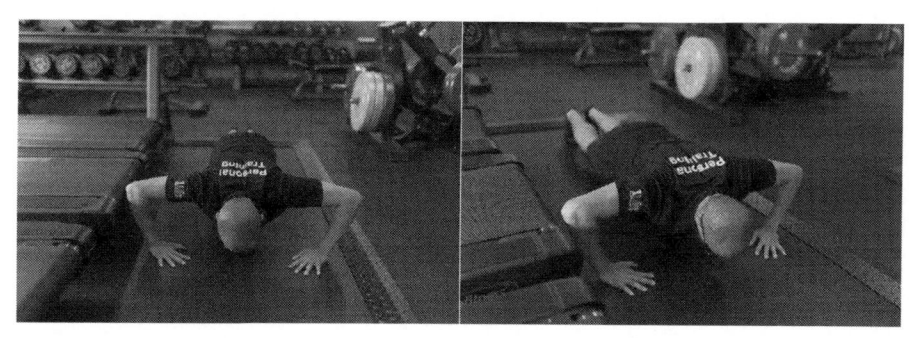

-Not going down enough (your chest shoulder almost touches the floor)

-Not keeping your body straight (lifting the hips too much or sagging)

-Not pause at the bottom (this is not a mistake, but in an ideal rep the rhythm would be slow and controlled instead of rushing through the rep).

Alternatives

-Nothing can substitute a good pushup but doing chest press and DB bench press is good to target chest, triceps, and shoulders.

How would it feel?

A proper pushup would activate many muscles. In fact, as you lower down you will initially feel your triceps working the most, while as you go lower

Dips

Why

Dips is considered "the squat of the upper body." It works your triceps, chest, and shoulders as well as you core to stabilise your body throughout the movement.

I am a big fan of this exercise as you can work on your maximal strength by doing weighted dips (look at the picture) as well as your relative strength by performing them bodyweight for higher reps.

Muscles Worked

Chest, Triceps, Shoulders (anterior part mainly) and Core

Maximal strength is how much strength you have overall. Relative strength is how much strength you have compared to your bodyweight. Most exercises work just on one of those two. Weighted dips (and weighted pull ups) work both ot those two strength components

How

-Grab the bar with arms straight and push shoulder down (do not

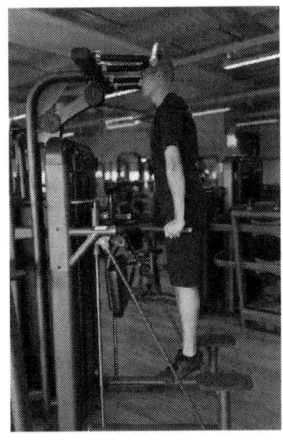

-Go down slowly and controlled at least to 90° angle (ideally lower).

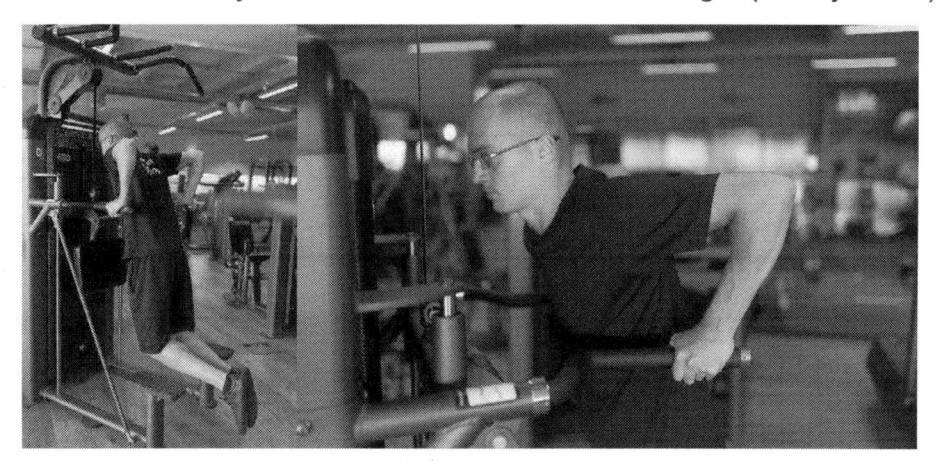

-Pause half a second at the bottom (at least) and

then push back up.

Regression/Progression

Before attempting dips, you would consider becoming strong in the pushups. Once you can do 15/20 pushups with perfect form it is time to think about doing dips as well (or just moving onto dips...that is up to you).

I would not recommend using the assisted dips machine as it does not work your core
(Assisted dips are a good tool to get stronger on your triceps, chest and shoulders, but I argue that is not the most effective way to learn how to do dips).

You can progress by increasing the range of motion and using a weighted belt. The progress in infinite in that sense.

Common Mistakes to Avoid

-Do not shrug (it might create shoulder pain if you perform the movement this way)

-Using momentum/Bouncing the rep (Pause at the bottom the get the most out of it)

-Cutting the Range of Motion short (At least 90° angle).

Alternatives

-Chest press (page 68) + Shoulder press (page 30)

-DB Chest Press (page 68)

-DB Overhead Press (page 77)

Pike Push ups

Why

Pike push-ups are a great exercise if you are looking to increase your shoulder strength exponentially!

It is the very first step to learn how to perform handstand pushups. In fact, Pike pushups will not only work your shoulders but also your triceps and core in a similar way that the handstand pushups do.

Muscles Worked

Shoulder (anterior part mainly), Triceps, Upper

Chest, and Core

How

-Go into a push up position.

-Lift your hips as high as you can while keeping your legs straight.

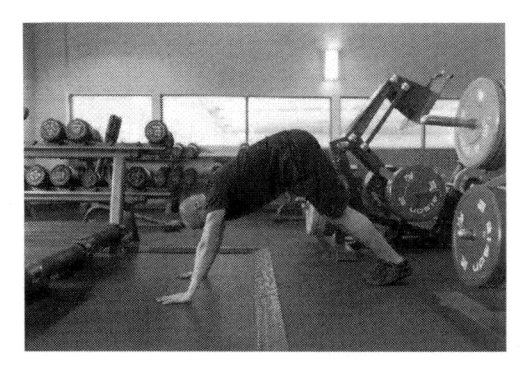

-From this position (your body should be in a reverse V position), bring your trunk down in a diagonal way. Your head should end up more forward than your hand positioning.

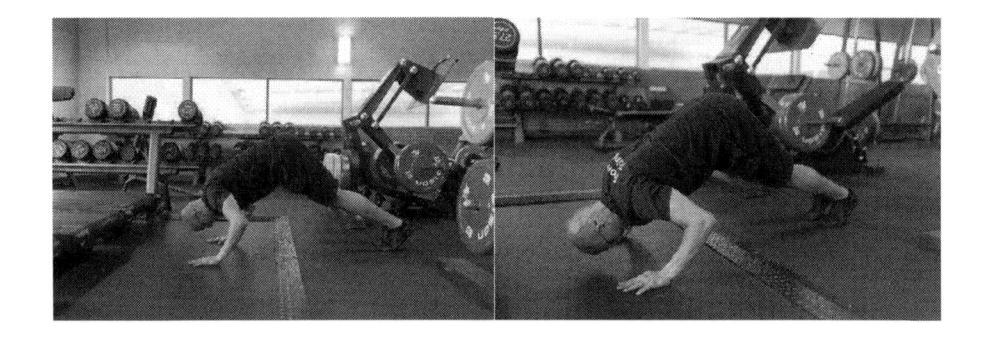

-Push back up into starting position.

Regression/Progression

-Change the angle and ROM.

You can start by having your feet and hands on the ground. Eventually you are going to lift your feet on an elevated surface to make it harder.

Moreover, you can also use some parallettes so you can go deeper down.

Common Mistakes to Avoid

-Not lifting your hips high enough. It takes a bit of mobility and coordination. I suggest you record your first attempts to evaluate your form.

-Up and down path. The path of the movement should be slightly diagonal. In fact, this mimic more the mechanics of a handstand pushups, and also put more overload on the shoulder. Moreover, it allows more range of motion, creating more time under tension for the shoulders.

Whether you train this movement for shoulder development or skill acquisition, the diagonal path is superior.

-Flaring out the elbows excessively.

How would it feel?

You will feel your shoulders doing the most part of the movement. However, you will feel your core working as to keep your body stable and firm throughout the movement.

PULL EXERCISES

Chin-ups

Why

Chin ups is an exercise that work your back and biceps (and core as well). If you get stronger in this exercise you will have benefits not only in terms of maximal strength but also relative strength. In fact, the stronger you are in chin ups the stronger you are compared to your bodyweight. To put is simple, you cannot be overweight and be strong in chin ups.

Muscles Worked

Back, Biceps and Core (to a lesser degree)

How

Start: Grab the bar shoulder-width apart (palms facing each other is the easiest version, so I highly suggest you start with that one) and start from the hanging position.

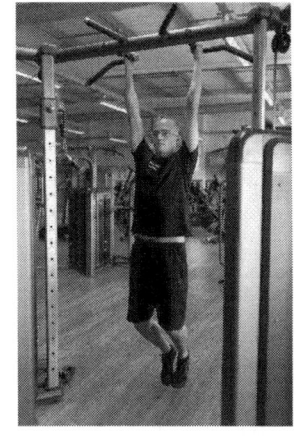

Finish: Upper chest touching the bar

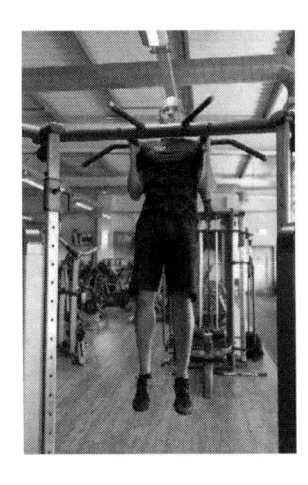

Note: Push shoulder down and think about bring your elbows down as you pull. The pull-up will seem easier as well as engaging your back more.

Pro Tip: Keep your feet in a dorsiflexed position (toes up). It helps create full body tension and elongate the spine.

Regression/Progression

Australian Rows (look next exercise to see how to do it).
Once you can do 10 of those, you will probably be able to do an eccentric chin up.

Eccentric chin ups mean jump/step, so you start with the chin over the bar. From there you hold the position on top of it for 3/5 seconds and then go down as slow as possible (up to 10 seconds). Once you master the "way down" of the chin-ups, you will be able to do a chin-up!

Once chin-ups become too easy (10+reps) might be time to use a weighted belt so you can overload it!

Elite athletes can load 50% of their body weight and perform 3/5 reps.

Alternatives

Lat Pulldown (page 44) and DB Pullover (page 87) are two good exercises that similarly target your back. However, some exercises are so good and effective that cannot be substituted. Chin-ups are one of those exercises.

The underhand version is probably the easiest for most people. You can also try the pronated grip (palms facing forward) to work more on your upper back, or the neutral grip (palms facing each other) that is easier on your elbow and shoulder joints.

Common Mistake to Avoid

-Cut the range of motion short (both on top, without having the chin over the bar and at the bottom, without fully elongate your arms)

-Protract your shoulders on top instead of being opened. By doing that you will not recruit the upper back muscles.

-Bringing your legs forward. By doing that you will activate more your core rather than your back.

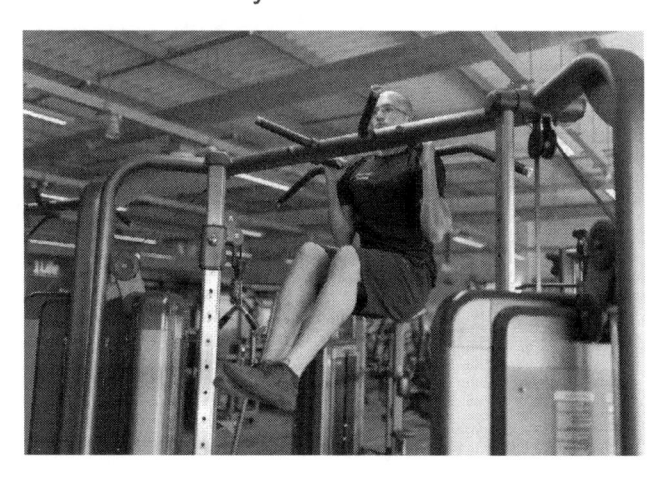

Inverted Rows

Why

It is a bodyweight movement that works your back and biceps. It is good to work on the back thickness and as a regression before doing pullups. Moreover, it is very easy to scale regardless of your starting fitness level.

By doing Australian Rows (or Inverted Rows, name it as you prefer it), you will feel tension in your whole body. In fact, it can be defined as reverse push-ups due to the core stability needed, and the nature of the movement.

Muscles Worked

Back, Biceps

How

Grab the bar slightly wider than shoulder-width apart

Keep your legs straight and think your body like a stick (from ankle to shoulders you must be completely straight, so make sure to squeeze your glutes and engage your core).

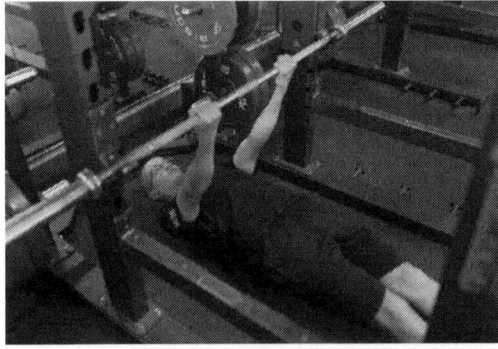

Pull yourself up with your sternum/lower chest touching the bar.

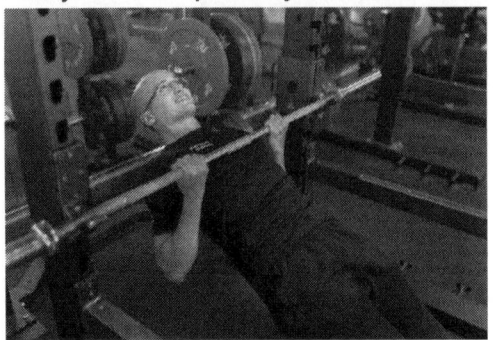

Come back down and do it again.

Regression/Progression

You can start by:

1) bend your knees with your feet on the floor

2) leg straight (like images above)

3) Leg elevated on a box

4) time to do chin-ups!

As a rule, once you can perform 10+reps it is probably time to step into the next progression

Common Mistakes to Avoid

-Rounding your shoulders on top instead of having your chest up. This is by far the most common mistake people do. It is usually lack of strength. If that is the case either find an easier variation or decrease the number of reps.

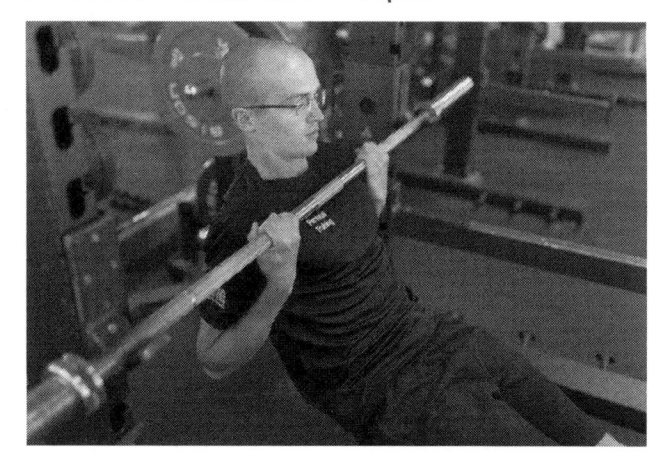

-Not having your hips extended throughout the movement (squeeze your glutes to make sure your hips are extended all the time)

-Not going all the way up (find an easier regression. If you cannot go all the way up with the knees bent, start by doing other exercises, and come back to this one in a few weeks)

-Touching the bar with the upper chest/neck or belly (adjust your feet positioning, backward or forward as to once you pull the lower chest touch the bar)

Alternatives

-DB Row (page 83)

-DB Pullover (page 87)

-Chin-ups (page 126)

-Lat Pulldown (page 44)

Ideally do DB Row as it is the same movement pattern, but other exercises as the ones mentioned works well.

CORE EXERCISES

Plank

Why

Plank is one of the foundations exercises you can do for your core. In fact, I would say this is the entry level for everyone (unless you are particularly overweight. In that case I would not recommend it). It works your core in a functional way as it has to resist to extend excessively. Moreover, it teaches you motor control and body awareness.

Muscles Worked

Core

How

-Put your elbows below your shoulders and keep your feet together.

-Think about your body as a straight line.

-Hold that position for as long as you can (one you can do 60" you can progress it into more difficult variations.

Regression/Progression

-You can start with your feet slightly wider to hold your balance easier.

-When you can do a 60" Plank you can bring your feet back, so the lever is longer. By doing this you will put more tension on your abs.

-Another progression would be to use the medicine ball on your elbows. You need to really squeeze your core to keep balance!

Common Mistakes to Avoid

-There is one big mistake that is the hip positioning. It does not have to be too high or too low as it can cause low back pain and it does not make this exercise effective.

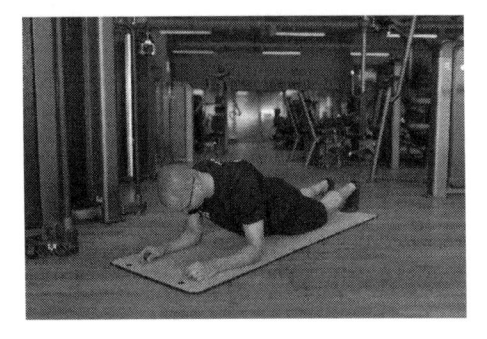

Hips too low

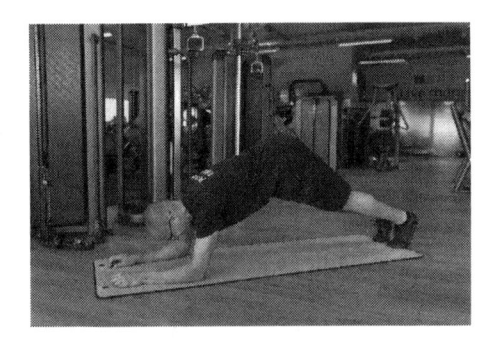

Hips too high

Note: In case you feel your low back in a plank stop. You are either holding it for too long and your body is compensating ì, or your technique is not right.

How would it feel?

If you have bever done it before you will feel a strong contraction on your core as you start. Moreover, you will also feel your shoulders and thigs working. After a few sessions you will feel it much less at first. The improvements will be very quick in this exercise if done consistently for more than 3x/ week.

Side Plank

Why

Side Plank is an amazing exercise for your obliques. By doing this you not only develop a strong and functional trunk that will assist you in many daily movements, but also you decrease the likelihood of low back pain. In fact, it works you obliques and Quadratus Lumborum, a deep muscle of your abs which strength is inversely correlated to low back pain the stronger, the less knee pain you will have).

Moreover, studies showed that it has an impact in decreasing knee injury. In fact, having a strong core allows your body to resist to sport contacts and be more resilient.

Muscles Worked

Obliques

How

-Lift yourself, with elbows and the outside of one foot touching the floor.

-The elbow should be just below the shoulder, while your feet should be one on top of the other.

-Lift your hips by creating a perfect diagonal line.

-Face your body directly in front of you and keep your non-working hand on the side.

You will feel a strong contraction on the side of your trunk as well as your shoulders. The first few times you will be shaky as soon as you get into position. Over time it will get easier and easier.

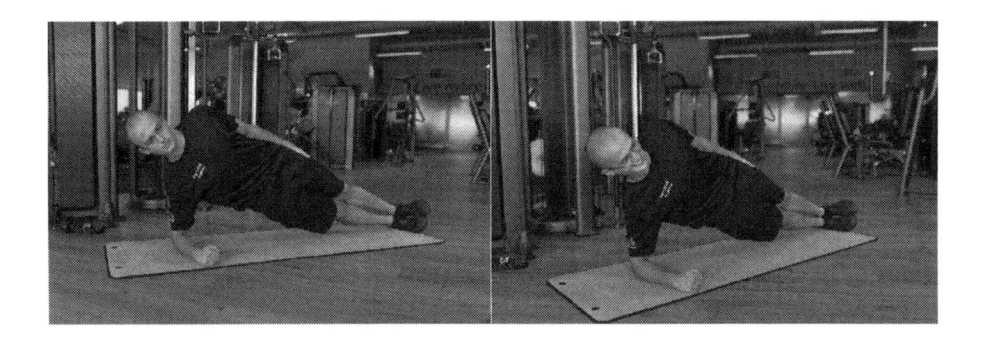

Regression/Progression

*Progress each step once you can do 60"

-You can start by doing it on your knees.

-Then go into the normal side plank.

-Then, you can lift the non-working leg as high as you can (it will

work the outside of your glutes too).

Common Mistakes to Avoid

-Hip positioning. This is the only mistake you can do when doing side plank, assuming your starting position is correct.

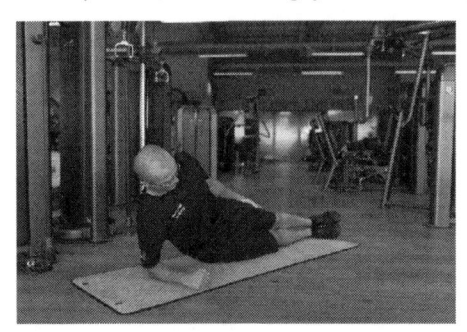

Make sure not to have it too high or too low (recording yourself or having someone to see how you do it can be beneficial at first)

How would it feel?

You will feel a strong contraction on the side of your trunk as well as your shoulders. The first few times you will be shaky as soon as you get into position. Over time it will get easier and easier.

LOWER BODY BOX

Pistol Squat

Why

It Is a great unilateral movement that will improve your athleticism, coordination, proprioception. It works your quadriceps and glutes. Moreover, by performing exercise as this one you will avoid having imbalances in between legs.

Muscles Worked

Quads and Glutes

How

-Stand on one leg with a box knee-height just behind you.

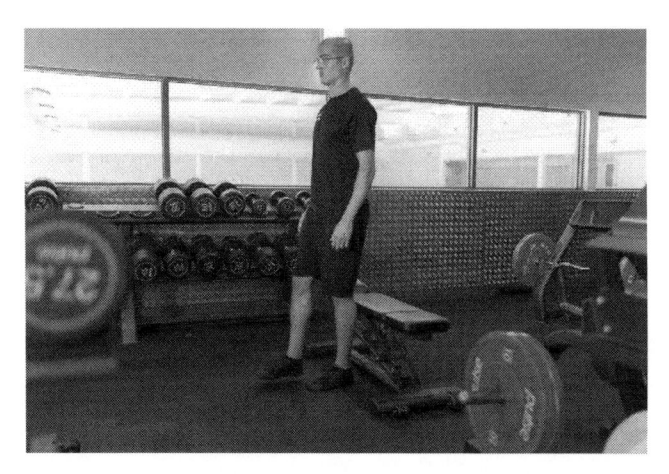

-Go slowly and controlled down until you sit on the box (while keeping balance only on one leg).

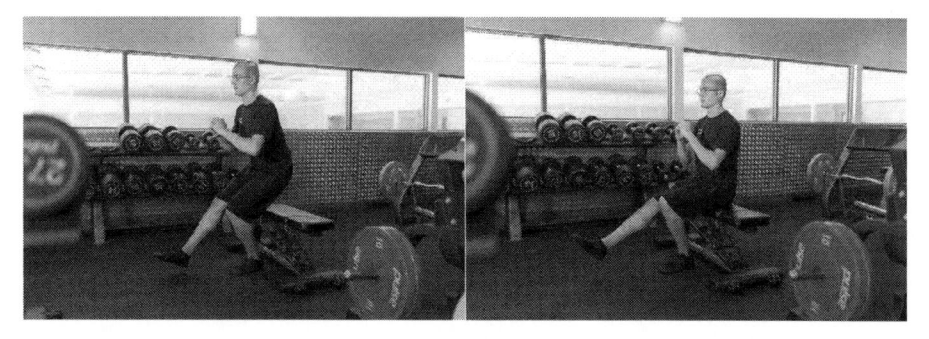

-Stand back up while using only

that one leg.

Regression

-Use a higher box if you have one. It will ensure that the range of motion is shorter, so the exercise will be slightly easier.

-Go down with one leg, but if you struggle to stand back up using only one leg, you can stand up with two legs.

-If instead you struggle with balance, you can use a stick to help yourself. Overtime you will put less and less pressure on that, so the assistance will be limited.

Progression

-Remove a box if you want to increase the range of motion. The lower you go the more you will work your glutes, adductor as well as ankle mobility.

-If you want to overload the movement you can start by holding a dumbbell in front of you.

Alternatives

-Bulgarian Split squat (page 138)

-Lunges (Page 113)

How would it feel?

At first you might struggle to go down while keeping the balance. It is normal and within two to three sessions you should be able to master it. The way will be more difficult, but if you have been doing strength training for a few months, it should not take too long before you can push yourself up with only one leg.

Bulgarian Split Squat

Why

As the Single leg squat mentioned above, this unilateral movement works quads and glutes.

Moreover, it will stretch your hip flexor of the rear leg. Due to modern lifestyle the hip flexors tend to be weak and tight, so this exercise will help you fixing this problem.

Muscles Worked

Glutes and Quads

How

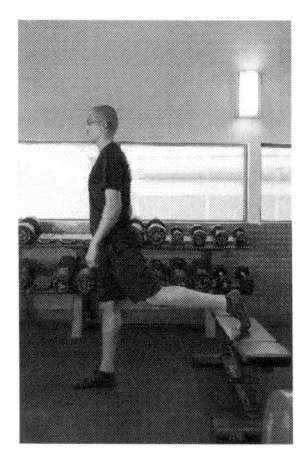

- Go slowly down until your hips are below your knees.

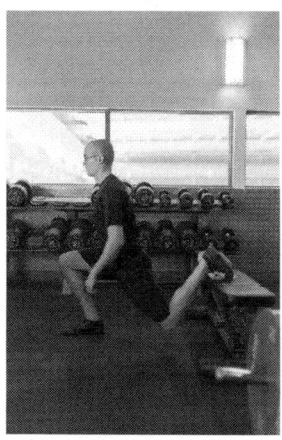

-Push back up.

Regression/Progression

-If you want to make it easier simply decrease the range of motion until you feel comfortable going lower.

-If you want to make it harder start by holding dumbbells on your side. Overtime aims to increase the load (make sure not to cur the range of motion short!)

Common Mistake to avoid

The only mistake people tend to do is to have a stance too short or too big. Find the right foot positioning so when you go down your hips are below your front knee, as well as your front knee a bit over your toes.

Alternatives

-Based on how you incline your trunk, you target more specific muscle. If you keep your trunk upright, you will work more your quads, while if you lean forward a bit, you'll feel it more on your glutes.

How would it feel?

At first you will struggle with the balance. After that it will be one of the most rewarding exercises you can do to develop a strong and athletic lower body. Unlike squats and lunges, you will also feel a stretch on the hip flexor of the non-working leg. It will be uncomfortable at first, but very useful as it will diminish the likelihood of back pain and knee pain in the long run.

Glute Bridge

Why

This movement is like hip thrust, so it will work your glutes and hamstrings. It is an excellent movement for your posterior chain. Moreover, the learning curve is very short, and pretty much everyone can start doing it.

Muscles Worked

Glutes and Hamstrings

How

-Lay on the floor with chest up

-Bend your knees and feet hip-width apart flat on the floor.

-Push the glute up by squeezing your glutes.

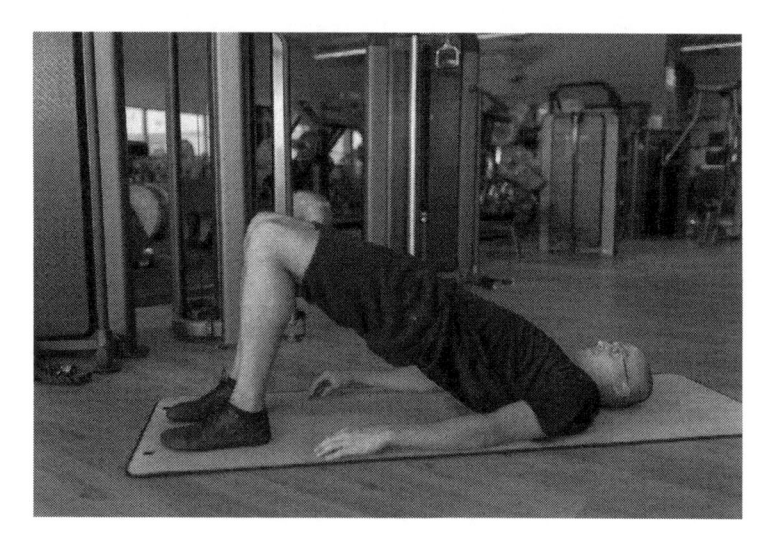

-Hold the position on top for a second.

-Come back down (lose the tension by letting the plates touch the bar) and go again.

Regression/Progression

- To make it more challenging use a barbell or a sandbag on your pelvis.

- If that is still too difficult you can start by doing it bodyweight (or try single leg for a more difficult progression).

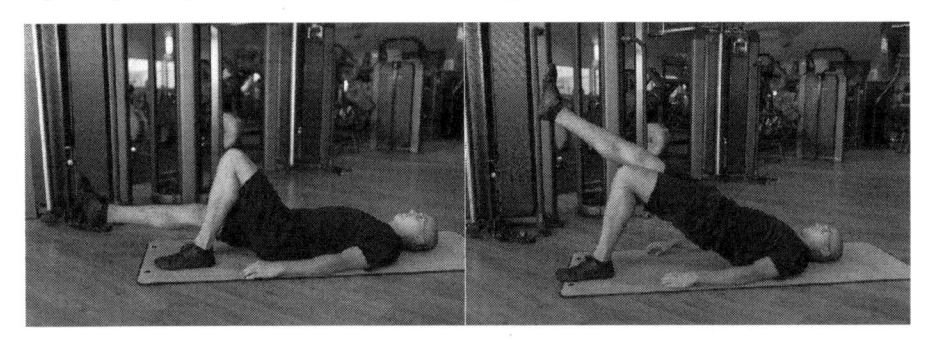

-To make it more challenging simply increase the load overtime.

Common Mistake to Avoid

-Bounce through reps. Do not use momentum between reps

-Not Locking the glutes on top of the movement (from the side you should be a perfect diagonal line from your shoulders to your knees).

Alternatives

-Hip thrust (page 107)

-RDL (page 110)

How would it feel?

It would feel like a Hip Thrust, but with more work on the upper glutes. Easy to learn and to progress. You should not face any difficulties in doing these movement

Stability Ball Leg Curl

Why

It is a great exercise to target your hamstrings. Unlike exercises such as RDL and Hip Thrust that target your hamstring by extending the hips, this exercise will work your hamstrings by flexing the knee.

Muscles Worked

Hamstrings

How

-Put your heels on the ball and lay on the ground like when you perform Glute Bridge.

-By keeping your hip up and glutes engaged, move the ball back and forth slowly and controlled.

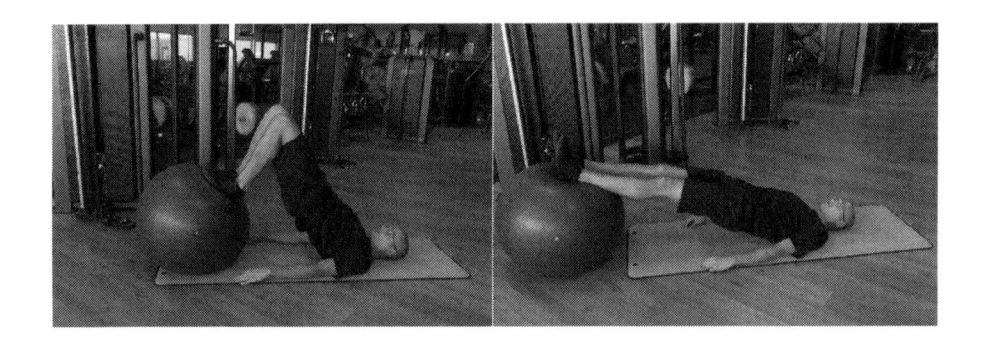

Regression/Progression

-You can start by performing this movement with both feet on the ball and move slowly.

-Once it gets easy, try to use it only one leg on the ball. It is going to be challenging at first, but then you will get used to it, get the proper balance, and perform it easily.

Common Mistake to Avoid

-Bounce through reps. Do not use momentum between reps

-Not Locking the glutes on top of the movement (from the side you should be a perfect diagonal line from your shoulders to your knees).

Alternatives

-Hip thrust (page 107)

-RDL (page 110)

How would it feel?

You will feel it on your hamstring as you bring the ball farther from you. Then focus on bringing your heel close to your glutes (imagine doing a bicep curl with your leg).

For more stability leave your arms next to your trunk in contact with the floor. This way you can focus more on your legs.

NOTE: to get the most out of it go slowly when lengthening your leg so you can feel your hamstring working more. Mind-muscle connection is key!

BULLETPROOFING EXERCISES

This section is extremely useful if you:

-Play sports and must put an effort in avoid injuries

-Have joint pains and want to improve the situation but you do not know how

-Want to bulletproof your body to avoid injuries

ANKLE

Tibialis Raise

Why

-It works the tibialis, a muscle attached at the front of your tibs. It is the first line of the defense for knees.

-It prevents shin splits, so very useful for runner and non.

-It allows you to decelerate faster as it works the exact movement pattern that we do when we decelerate.

How

-Stand with your glute touching the wall and slightly leaning forward to start.

-Find a comfortable distance (usually two feet from the wall is a good starting point).

-Flex your foot up while keeping your knees straight

*When flexing your foot up apply pressure with your heel to the ground.

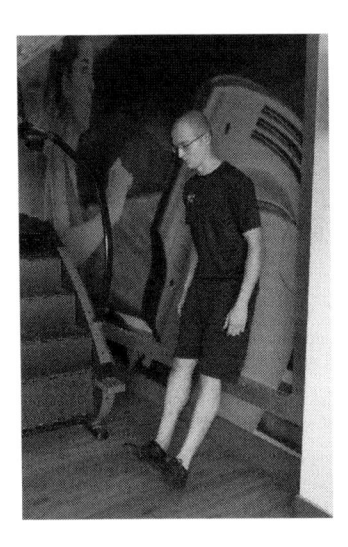

-Keep that position for 2 seconds while squeezing up your foot (you should really feel the muscle in front of your tibs working)

Go back into starting position with foot fully relaxed on the ground.

Regression/Progression

The closer your feet to the wall the easier it gets. The farther from the wall, the more challenging.

Common Mistakes to Avoid

-Bending your knees and not having your legs straight

-Not lifting your foot completely (you will probably need to stand closer to the wall to get the full range of motion)

Calf Raises

Why

Training your calves is very important to avoid Achilles tendon pain and to protect your knees when landing from a jump. Whether you are an athlete or not, you should be doing calf raises at least once a week as it also avoids plantar fasciitis, very common for old or overweight people.

How

-Stand tall with feet hip with apart.

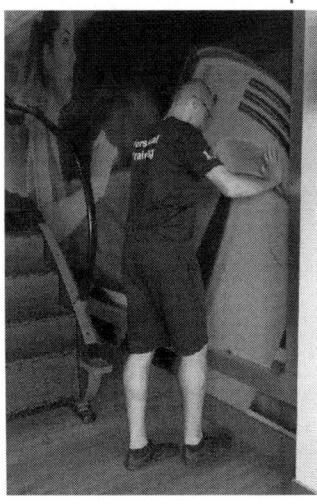

-Lift your heels as high as you can.

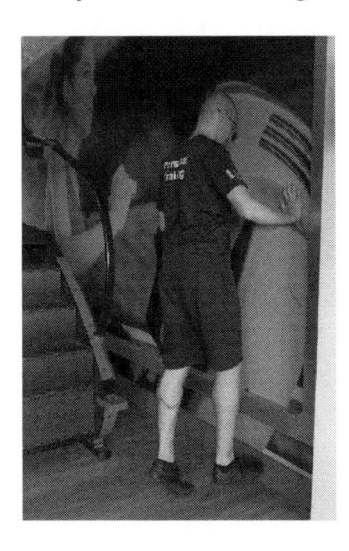

-Hold that position for a couple of second

-Go back into starting position

Regression/Progression

You regress it by holding your hand onto a wall if you lack balance.

You progress it either doing it single leg or using weight (dumbbells on your hands or barbell on your back).

Common Mistake to avoid

   -Incomplete range of motion/ Not going all the way up.

   -Not squeezing on top/Bounce back down.

   -Not having you knees straight when doing it but bending them.

KNEE

Patrick Step-up

Why

working in a short range of motion is important to get blood flow to their area, especially knees, before doing other movements such as squats and lunges.

Studies showed how this exercise helps athletes not only to perform better (it is unilateral, so more "sport specific"), but also to avoid and decrease the likelihood of Patellar tendons and ACL/MCL tears.

It works the VMO, the teardrop muscle above the knee. This muscle is the first one to contract when the knee is under pressure. So, it makes sense to strengthen it for both longevity and athleticism.

How.

-Stand on a step and balance on one leg

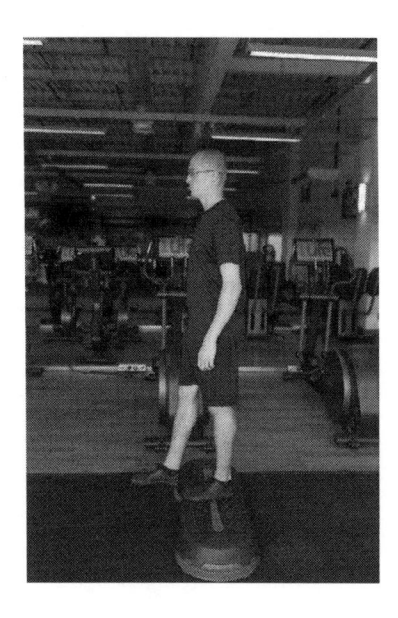

-Slowly go down with the other leg until the heel touches the floor.

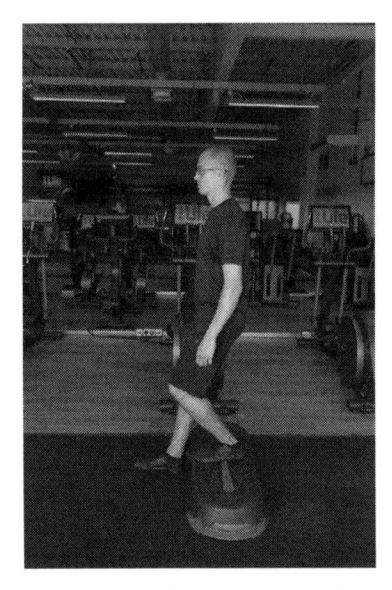

-At that point push back up with the working leg. Bonus tips:

-Make sure the non-working leg is straight

-Go down slowly

-The knee of the working leg must be aligned with the foot and not caving in.

Regression/Progression

-To make it easier use a smaller step (or not use one at all)

-To make it harder elevate the steps' height or use dumbbells/barbells to load the movement.

Common Mistakes

-Sitting back with the hips instead of driving them forward (this would put less tension on your knees. With this step up we want to overload the knee and the muscle around it)

-Losing balance (focus on three contact points: your heel, big toes and below your pinkie...these three points must apply pressure on the ground)

Reverse Nordic Curl

Why

Reverse Nordic is a great exercise to strengthen your quads, especially the rectus femoris. The rectus femoris is the deepest muscle in our things that exercises such as squat and lunges do not target directly.

Moreover, it works the connective tissue (tendons, ligaments, and fascia) around the knees as at the bottom of the range those tissues are stretched completely, and from that position they have to push the body back up (it can be seen as a loaded stretching). For athletes it is an important exercise as it prevents the likelihood of quads strains.

For non-athlete it is also important as it work the hip flexor in a position that we are rarely in. By siting all day, the hip flexor tends to be weak and tight. This exercise reverses that effect.

Being able to perform Reverse Nordic full range pain free means that you have:

-resilient quads on an extreme range of motion under load.

-great knee and patellar tendon tolerance. Knees are very healthy to be in full extension without pain.

-elite ankle mobility and capacity (dorsiflexion).

-great core strength, especially if you can keep your pelvis neutral as you go down.

How

-Start with your knee and feet on the floor.

-Put your hands on the side of your body.

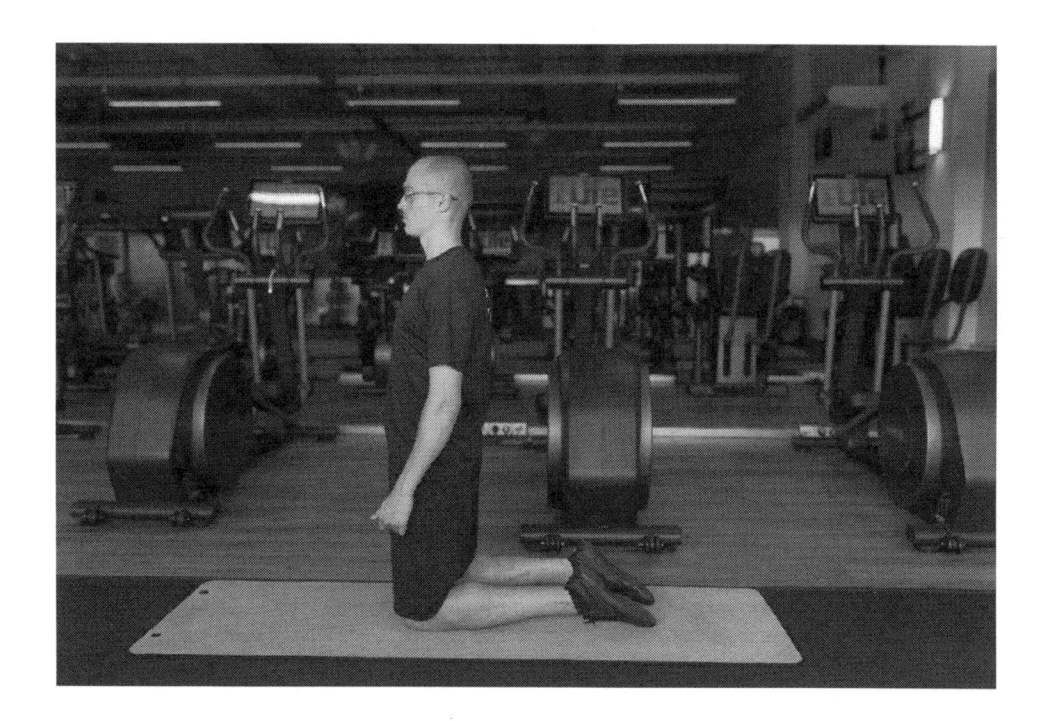

-Lower down as low as possible (ideally with your upper back touching the ground). And perform the movement in a slow and controlled manner.

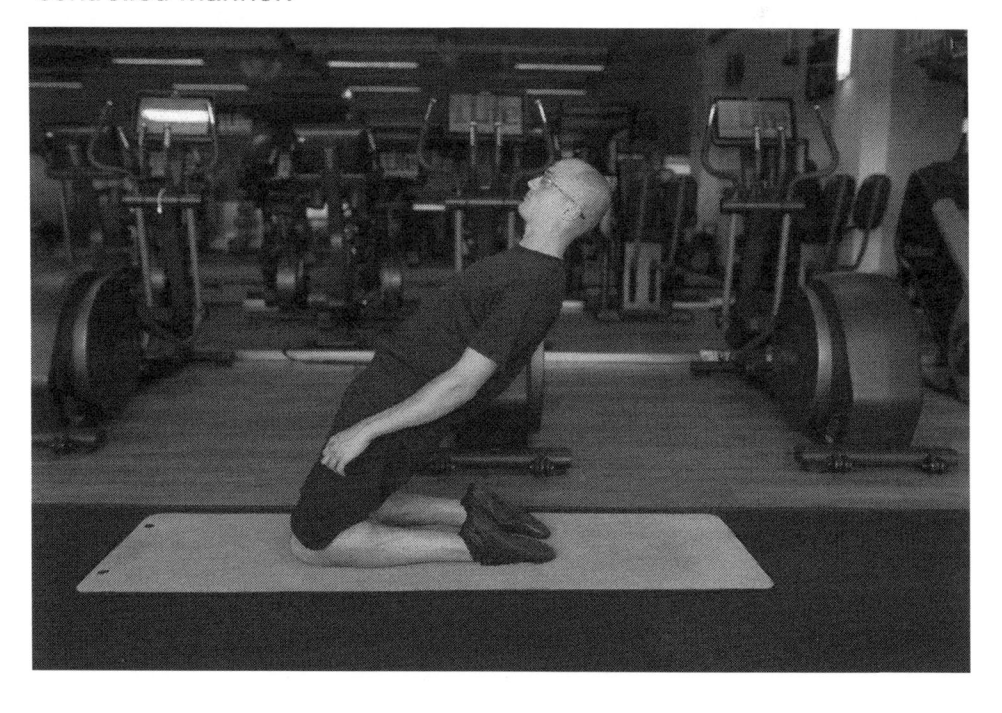

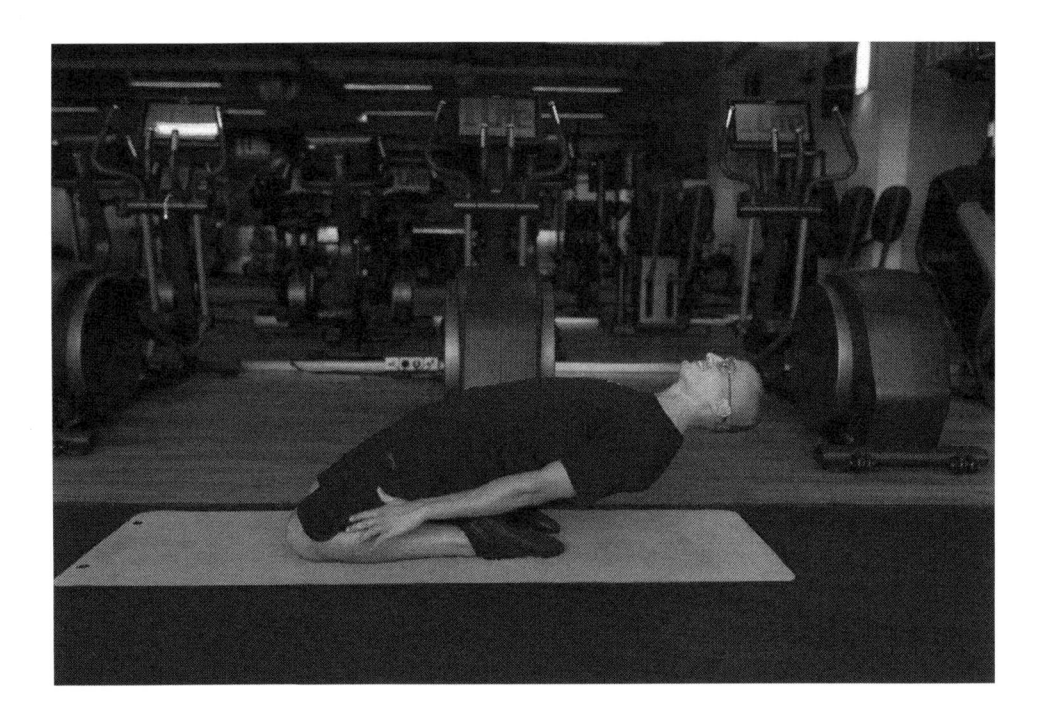

-From there, push back up keeping your glutes contracted (so you do not bend the hips). If that is too difficult you can put your arms in front of you (as I did in the last 2 reps).

Once a week for 2/3 sets of 5 reps is more than enough. Doing it more than once a week I think would be too demanding for the connective tissue around the knee.

Regression/Progression

You can start by putting a support below your feet to make it easier.

Once the normal version (the one showed in the video) gets easy, you can:

1) put your hands crossed your chest.
2) pick a weight and hold it on your chest.
3) keep increasing the weight.

Common Mistakes

-Bending at the hips. Keep your pelvis neutral is key to engage the core and get the most out of it. If you cannot do it yet that is fine. Just work on a range of motion in which you can keep it that way.

-Going too fast without control (especially the way down is key to go slow!)

How would it feel?

At first you feel a good stretch on your quads, and you might not feel comfortable all the way down (and that's ok!). Some people experience cramp on their feet in the first session as their feet have never experienced that position (well, we did when we were child but then due to modern shoes and lifestyle, we never explore that range of motion).

SPECIAL OFFER: do you feel like you need an extra help and accountability for your fitness journey? Go to **avfitness99.wixsite.com** or DM me on **Instagram- avfitness99-** and see the different possibilities that you can get from Online Coaching.

PERSONALISED PLAN

Tailored 4 weeks plan based on your goals and gym frequency

-Free Zoom Consultation

-4 weeks plan

-Video Tutorial for Each Exercise

MONTHLY COACHING
Perfect for people serious to get fit

-Free Zoom Consultation

-4 weeks plan

-Video Tutorial for Each Exercise

-Nutritional Guidelines

-Training Check 2x/weekly

-Answer to any question within 24 hours

ELITE COACHING Full accountability for training /lifestyle

-Free Zoom Consultation

-4 weeks personalised plan

-Video Tutorial for each exercise

-Nutritional advice

-Lifestyle advice

-Daily text for workout

-Daily text for diet/lifestyle

-24/7 Support and accountability

-2 Zoom individualized HIIT Workout a month

Now let's go back to the book!

*The offer might change overtime. Look at my Instagram or website to stay in touch

with the most recent updates.

AVFITNESS99

SCAN ME

Nordic Curl

Why

Reverse Nordic is a great exercise to strengthen your hamstrings (and lower back and calves). This exercise is often used by athletes to avoid injuries/strains in the hamstring and knees. It can also be a good exercise for non-athletes as it is quite common for adults to pull the muscle at the back of the leg when running.

Moreover, it works the connective tissue (tendons, ligaments, and fascia) around the knees, making it an amazing exercise to bulletproof your lower body.

How

-Lock your feet on a bar and go with your knees on the floor.

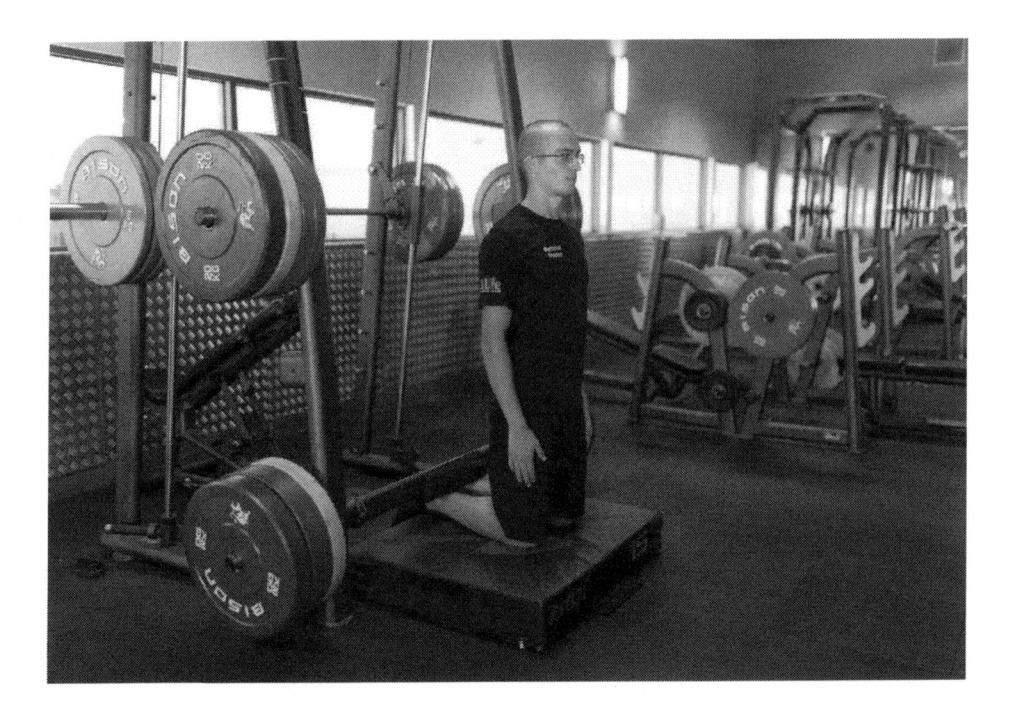

-From this position lower down as slow as possible until your body is almost touching the floor.

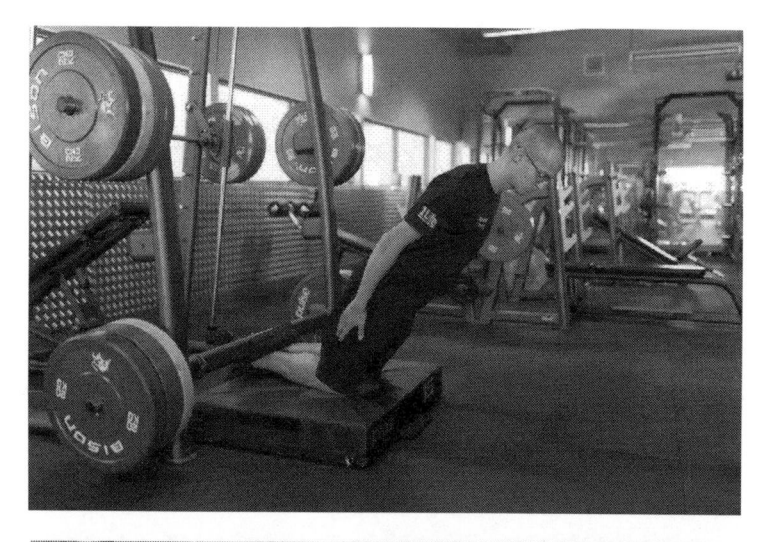

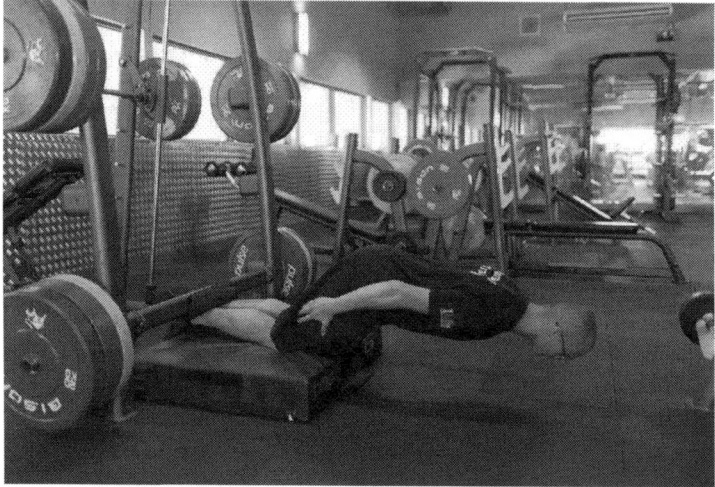

-Then use your hands to help yourself push back up into starting position and go again (eventually you will be able to come back into starting position without using your hands, as in the image below).

Regression/Progression

-To regress it you can use a box in front of you as the range of motion would be shorter. Moreover, you can also bend at the hips (slightly though, do not exaggerate it) to make it a bit easier.

-To progress it you might try to come back up just using the power of your hamstrings. Then, you might also try to overload it by holding a plate on your chest (this would be very advanced, and it will probably take you years to get to this level).

Common Mistakes to Avoid

-Do this exercise if you are a complete beginner.

I would highly recommend you spend 2/3 months doing other exercises such as RDL or Leg Curl before attempting this exercise.

-Going too fast down.

The main point of the exercise is to go slowly down as the hamstring is strong enough to control your body. If you go fast down with little or no time under tension, this exercise is not as effective as it would be.

-Bending the hips too much.

You will probably need to bend them the first few sessions (and in the future, most likely). However, your goal is to try to be as straight as possible from your knees to your shoulders.

Alternatives

RDL (page 110)

Leg Curl (page 57)

How would it feel?

You will probably feel like your hamstring is pulling at first. Take this movement very slowly into your routine. I would say that this exercise works your hamstring like no other, so if you are serious about avoiding strains and pull muscle, please do it!

ATG Split Squat

Why

ATG split squat is a great lower body exercise as it works:

-ankle mobility (the better you can dorsiflex the less likely of ankle and knee injury you have).

-knee flexion (by going to an extreme long range aka knee over toes and full coverings of calves with the hamstring, you allow the synovial fluid on your knees to go through your connective tissue, making your tendons and ligaments more resilient).

-hip flexor mobility and strength (the hip flexor of the back leg is stretched under load. Stronger and mobile hip flexor reduce the likelihood of low back pain). The more capacity you have to get into those deep ranges the more bulletproof and pin free you will be able to move your body

-avoid imbalances between legs as it is a unilateral movement. If you are a beginner, it is great to start doing unilateral movements to avoid imbalances between limbs. All resistance machines work your legs bilaterally, so incorporating from the very beginning ATG Split Squat will benefit you immensely!

How

-find a stance that allows you to:

1) fully cover your hamstring with calves, and heel touching the glutes
2) keep body straight
3) Back knee does not touch the floor

Move up and down slowly and controlled.

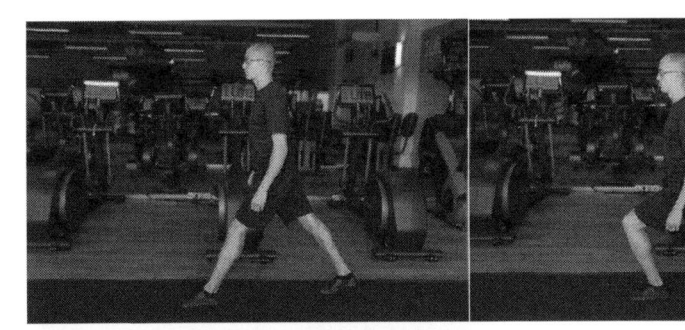

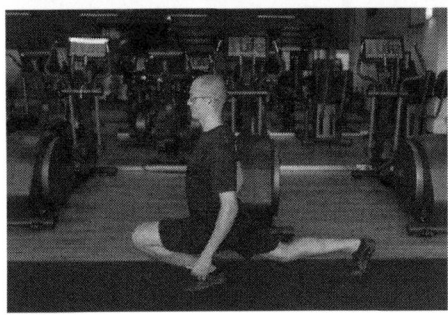

Also:

-Make sure to hold a second or two at the bottom

-Keep your foot flat on the step/floor at all times (do not elevate your toes once you push back up into starting position)

Regression/Progression

1) Start with a box in front of your feet
2) do it bodyweight without a box
3) hold dumbbells
4) have a bar on your back
5) have a bar in front, like front squat (as showed)

Alternatives

There are many exercises that you can do that works and address similar movements, such as Squats and Lunges. Personally, I do not think that you can find a better strength exercise that works your lower body mobility as the ATG Split Squat.

Common Mistakes

-Leaning forward. (By doing this you will not extend the hip flexor of the back leg. Get into this position is crucial for having fluidity in movement as well as having good posture and reduce low back pain)

-Losing balance (You can start by holding a stick, but overtime being aware of your body while doing this exercise will benefit you)

-Not pausing at the bottom (Bouncing back to squeeze more reps and/or lifting more weight

will benefit your ego, not your body…. Pause at the bottom, embrace the rep, and then push back up).

How would it feel?

Imagine a Bulgarian Split squat (page 138) …. but deeper. That's' it.Usually, people feel a nice stretch in their hip flexor and a good feeling on their knees afterwards. You will most likely experience something similar.

Pro tip: do it before Hip Thrust. I t will allow you for a better contraction once you close the movement.

HIPS
Knee Raises

Why

I like to think about this exercise as the opposite of the squat. In fact, we get into the same position final position

It works the hip flexor and rectus abdominis. Especially if you want to get fast (whether for short or long distances), hip flexor stretches, and size is one of the main differences between elite athletes and normal People.

How

-hang on a bar with arms straight.

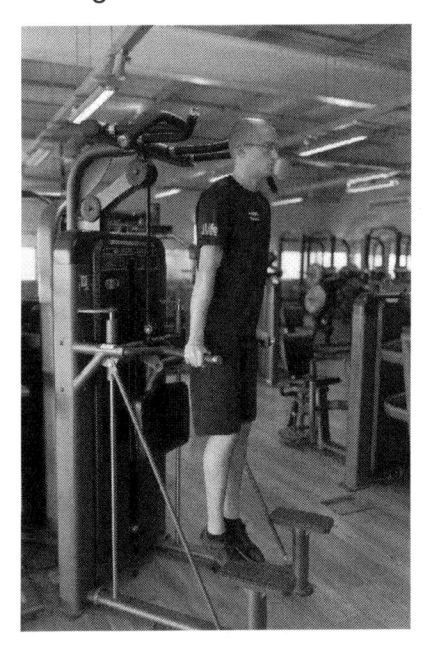

-Lift your knees as far as you can (drive your knees towards your chest)

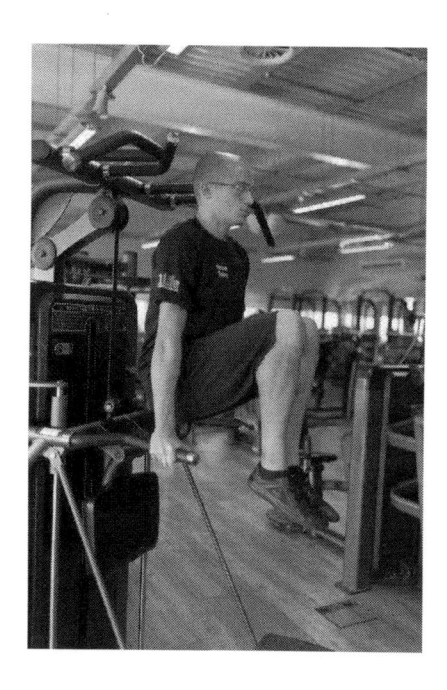

-Pause at the top for one second.

-come back slowly into starting position

Regression/Progression

You can progress it by doing it while lifting weights with your feet (simply put a dumbbell between your feet). A very good standard would be to perform 10/15 reps with a dumbbell equal to your 20% of bodyweight.

Alternatives

As an alternative you can use the dip bar to do it (it will work your shoulder and arms too).

Or you can do it isometrically on the floor. Sit with your legs straight in front of you and hands on the side. Lift your glutes so the only contact points with the ground will be your hands and your heels. Overtime you will elevate your heels too. 20 seconds hold works well.

Common Mistakes

-Using momentum and swinging (by doing this you not only will not get many benefits but also you might expose your Low back to injuries)

-cutting the range of motion too short (at least 90° must be achieved)

How would it feel?

You should feel it more on your lower abs and hip flexors. When you squeeze it and pause on top, it is normal to have a burning Sensation in those areas (it means you are giving a new stimulus to the body...and overtime you'll adapt to it.!)

RDL (already mentioned previously)

Why

RDL, or Romanian Deadlift, is one of the best exercises for the posterior chain (hamstring and glutes, but also your back will work) It allows to work your hamstrings by extending the hip and working your glutes in a stretched position (unlike hip thrust, for example).

I would like to think about this exercise as a loaded stretch. In fact, the connective tissues are lengthened as you go down. From that position, where we are at our weakest, we must be able to exert strength.

It is a fantastic exercise to bulletproof your hamstrings as well as getting stronger.

How

-Keep your back straight.

-Grab the bar slightly wider than shoulder width (your grip should be just outside your knees).

-Knee slightly bent in a fixed position throughout the entire movement.

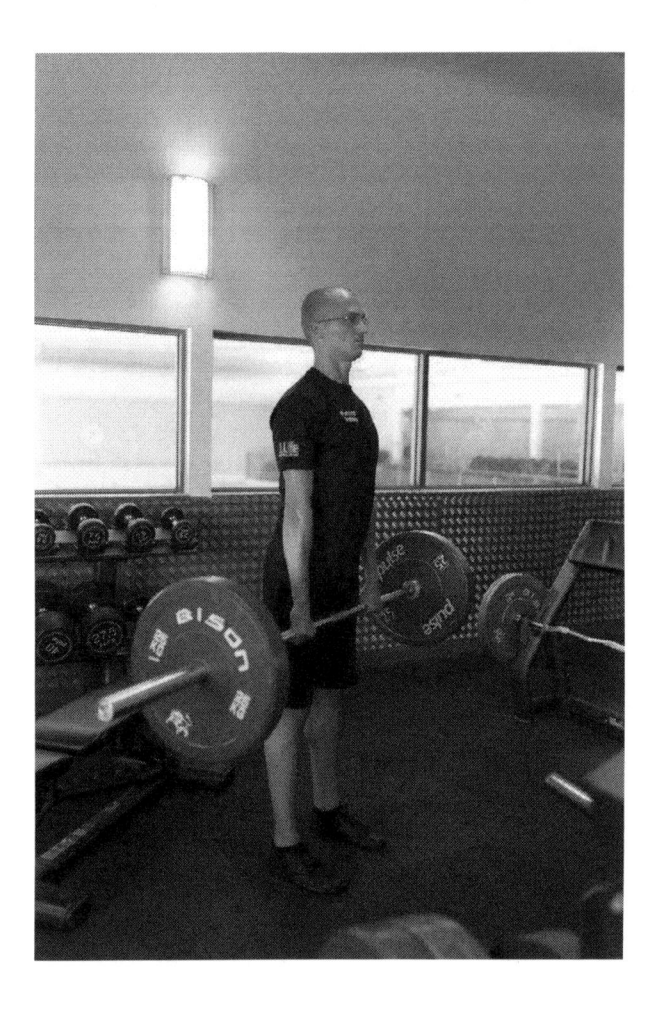

-Push the glutes back on the way down feeling a stretch on your hamstrings.

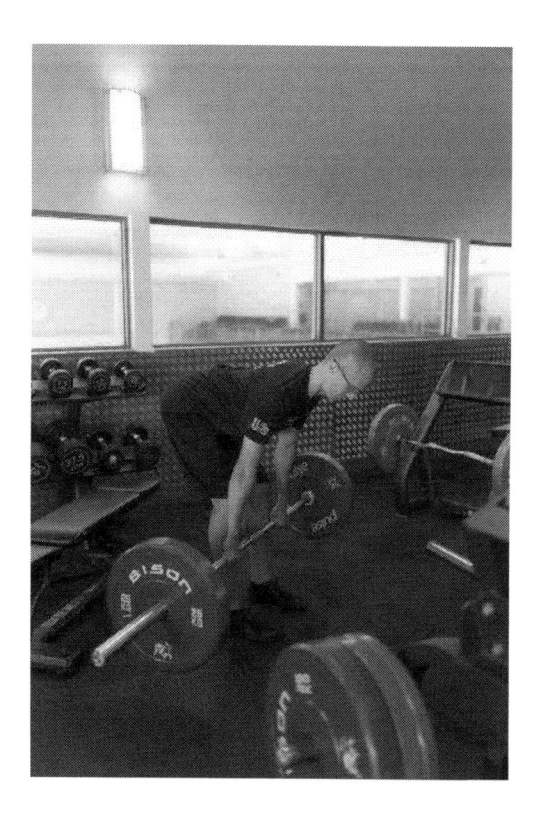

-Push back up hinging at the hips, pushing your feet (especially the heel) against the floor.

-Keep the bar close to your body throughout the entire movement

Regression/Progression

You can start with dumbbells, and then progress into a barbell.

A variation that you can do is to do it unilateral (requires more balance/coordination but give less possibility to overload).

A progression that you can try is to elevate your feet as to increase the range of motion.

Common Mistakes

Rounding your back (Rounding your spine is not wrong.... in fact, exercises such as Jefferson Curls are great to do. However, during RDL your back should be straight)

-let the barbell move forward (this will expose your low back as well as work less hamstrings and glutes)

Alternatives

As an alternative you might perform Leg Curl (go to page 57) or Nordic curl (go to page 159). These two exercises will not work your glutes unlike RDL but will target the hamstring.

The movement is going to be different (RDL works the hamstring by extending the hips, while those two works the hamstring by flexing the knee), but the result aka muscle activation, is going to be similar.

How would it feel?

As you go down, you will feel a nice stretch on your posterior chain. Once you push the barbell back up, you will feel the glutes helping to close the movement. You might also feel it on your back and grip.

If you do not feel it on your glutes when you push the bar up (but only in your hamstrings), once you push the bar back up, focus on pushing with your heels on the floor rather than your entire foot. This should do the magic!

Instead, if you feel it on your low back, chances are that you are going to low according to your mobility and strength. For most people going just below the kneecap it more than enough to get results.

It is an intense exercise, so plan it into your training accordingly.

SHOULDERS

Shoulder injuries are common for many people. The top three categories are:

-Gym goers that do lots of punishing exercises and neglect some pulling.

-Athletes that throw regularly.

Normal people that due to the nature of their job (scaffolding or construction, working at the desk all day etc. etc.) might have use too much or too little the shoulder joint.

DB External Rotation

Why

This simulates the exact opposite pattern of throwing. The idea behind it is that you want to be as strong in this exercise as in throwing something. By doing this you will not only avoid overused injury but also strengthen the muscle around your shoulder joint in the reverse of the movement.

How

-Sit on a bench with a leg bent on top (let's say the right one).

Grab a dumbbell with your right hand and put your right elbow on your right knee while keeping your trunk straight (chest up and nothing in the body moving)

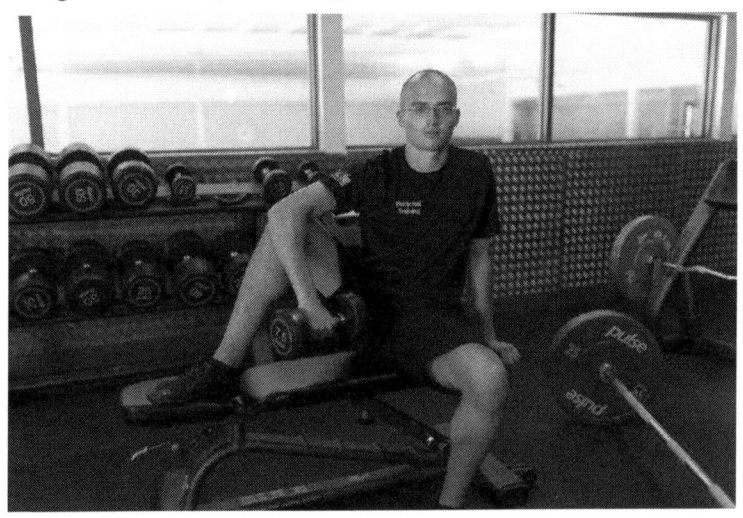

-From there you want to push the dumbbell up and back (the opposite movement of a throw) until the forearm is vertical to the ground.

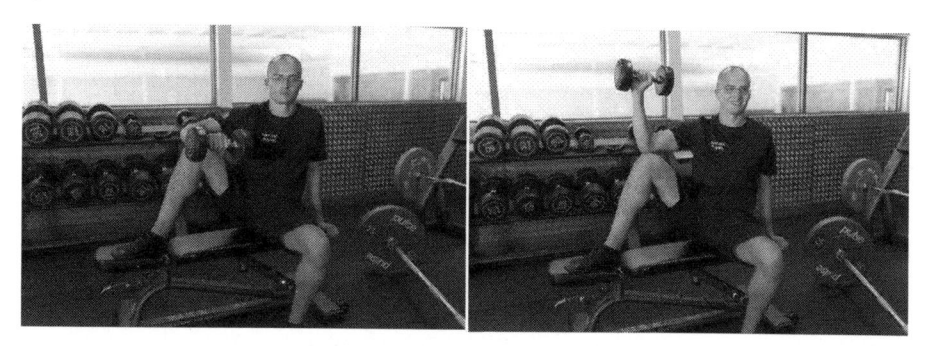

-Then lower down slowly and really fight to slow down the rep (same concept of Nordic Curl, page 159).

Regression/Progression

-10% BW for athletes/ fit people for 10+ reps must be the baseline.

Common Mistakes to Avoid

There are no common mistakes in this one.

Just make sure that there is no other motion in the body. You must isolate the movement and not create momentum with other part in your body.

Band Pull Apart

Why

This is a short-range movement that is going to target the posterior part of the shoulder as well as your upper back. It is very helpful to give blood flow to the area and heal your connective tissue, especially the rotator cuff, often overused by many gym-goers.

Most importantly, it helps to have a correct posture. As we sit all day we tend to hunch. By doing this movement we open our chest, and we work those muscles that are underused in our daily life activities.

How

-From a standing position, Grab a band shoulder width apart with your arms straight in front of your chest.

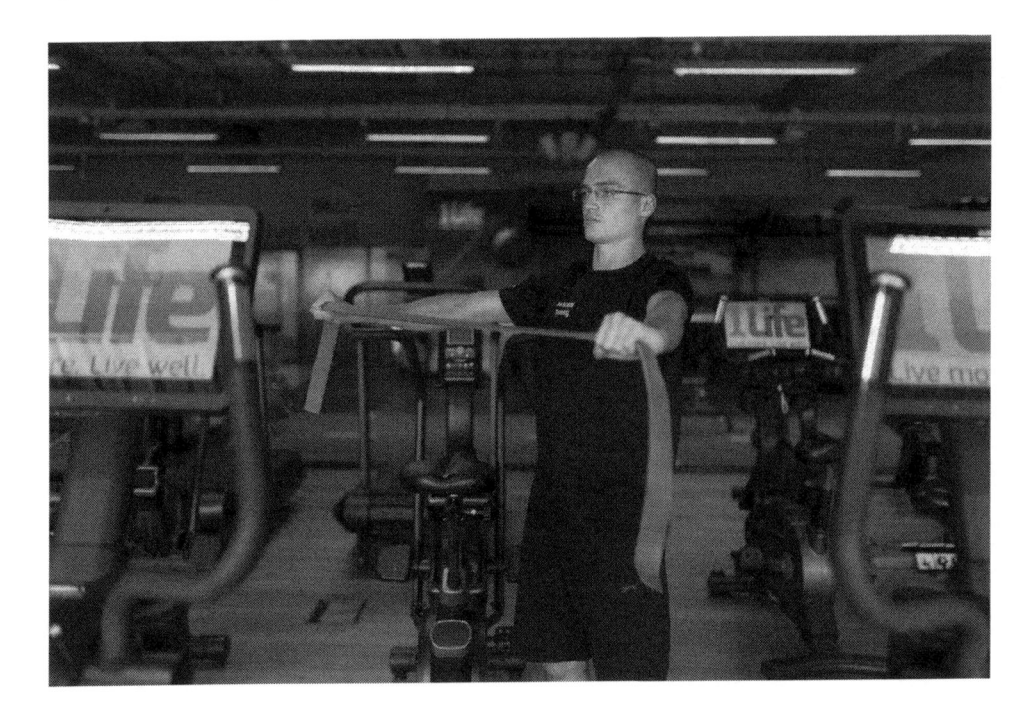

-From there, pull the elastic band to the side while keeping your arms straight.

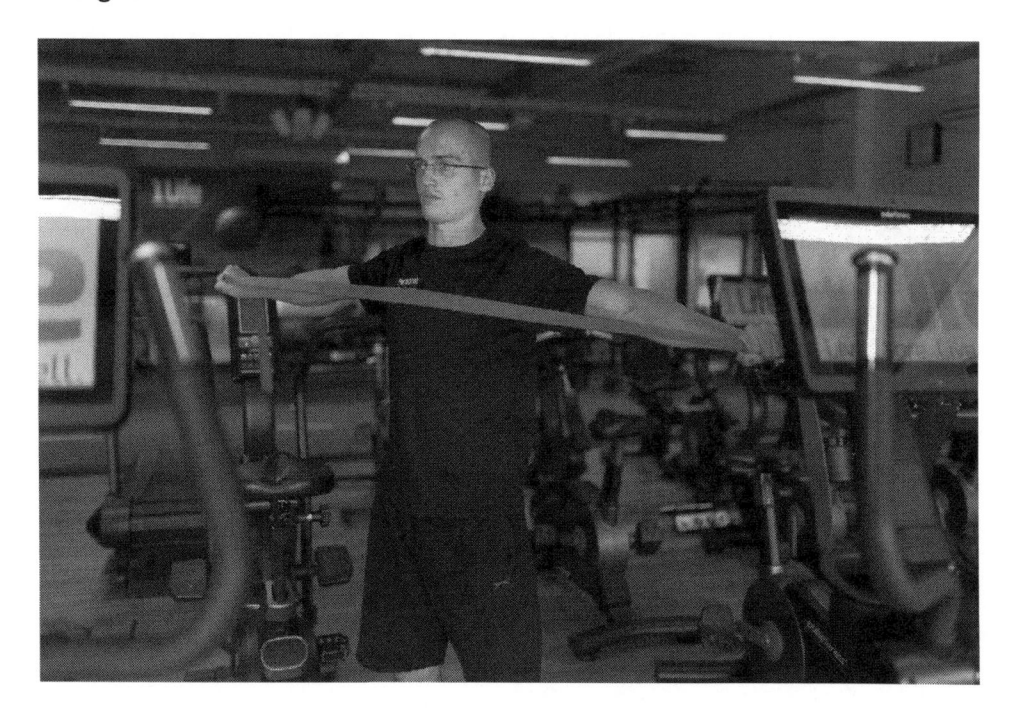

-Once you have your arms in line with your body, squeeze for 1" and go back into starting position (always keeping your arms straight)

Regression/Progression

-The wider you grab the band the easier it gets as the range of motion and intensity would decrease.

-The closer you grab it the harder the exercise

Common Mistake to Avoid

-Bent the elbows and wrist when performing it. Arms must be straight.

How would it feel?

You will feel a burning sensation in the muscle around out shoulder blades once you do more than 10/15 reps.

In this exercise I would suggest doing up to 20/25 reps.

BONUS PART

Healthy Lifestyle that will 10x your health (and fitness results)

Sunlight in the morning

Going outside within an hour of the waking time, even on cloudy days, showed terrific benefits for overall well-being, focus and mood throughout the day.

Many studies have been done on the importance and impact on sunlight, especially early in the morning…. Trust me, do not miss these benefits!

For example:

-Mood and emotional well-being

-Production of melatonin (then released at night) aka better sleep

-Hormones regulation

-Ability to Focus

-Immune function

-**Avoid Blue lights before going to sleep**

Sleep is extremely important for your well-being and for your fitness. Making sure that the quality of it is as high as possible is crucial (especially if you cannot sleep 8/9 hours at night)

-Do not eat until you are full

It does not matter what you eat; if you eat too much of food, you will be tired. Ideally you will not go above 85% of fullness to avoid that feeling

Meditate 10 minutes a day

This is a practice that can be done anywhere. It might be easier if you find a slot during the day to keep it as a habit (as soon as you wake up or before going to sleep are very good options)

You will definitely feel more centered, calm in stressful situations and in control of your actions if you stick with it for a few weeks.

Avoid alcohol

Many scientific studies proved that there are no benefits in alcohol consumption. Studies showed that even modest consumption predispose people to more stress and be less resilient overall.

"Alcohol is the only drug where if you don't do it, people assume you have a problem" cit. Chris Williamson

Where to find me

Website:

Instagram: avfitness99

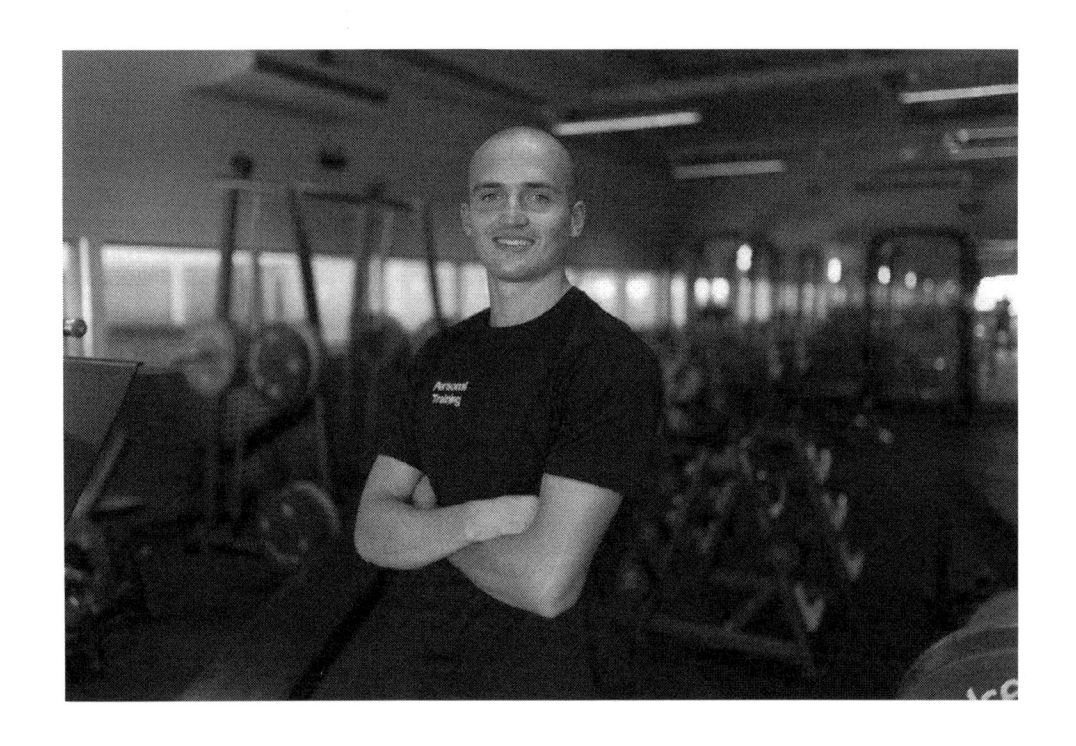

ABOUT ME?

Growing up, I always have had a strong passion for football. Wanting to excel physically in every area, I understood the importance of training (outside the football pitch) to prevent injuries and improve my athleticism. In the last 3/4 years I spent thousands of hours reading, listening, and watching experts in the industry give their ideas and tips on fitness. At least 1 hour of my day (almost every day) is always spent in learning from the best in the industry. This helped enhance my athleticism as well as in this book I tried to summarise the teaching points from the fitness gurus that I learnt in those years.

2 years ago, I became a Personal Trainer, and since then I spent hundreds of hours on the gym floor and training people 1-on-1 and in classes. By doing this I had thousands of different feedbacks about every exercise. Asking how they felt during a given exercise, what

muscle did they feel the most and seeing how my teaching points changed their feelings of an exercise has been a crucial aspect in writing this guide!

I decided to write this easy guide with lots of exercises so peopl over 40, that.....right exercises for them.

Hopefully, you learnt (or are learning) how to perform those exercises step by step, memorising the main teaching points that helped hundreds of people already!

With lots of exercises so people over 40, that often are not sure how to start their fitness journey, have a clear idea on how to structure their sessions and how to perform the right exercises for them.

REFERENCES

- Cauza, E., Hanusch-Enserer, U., Strasser, B., Ludvik, B., Metz-Schimmerl, S., Pacini, G., Wagner, O., Georg, P., Prager, R., Kostner, K., Dunky, A. and Haber, P., 2005. The Relative Benefits of Endurance and Strength Training on the Metabolic Factors and Muscle Function of People With Type 2 Diabetes Mellitus. *Archives of Physical Medicine and Rehabilitation*, 86(8), pp.1527-1533.
- Gippini, A., Mato, A., Pazos, R., Suarez, B., Vila, B., Gayoso, P., Lage, M. and Casanueva, F., 2002. Effect of long-term strength training on glucose metabolism. Implications for individual impact of high lean mass and high fat mass on relationship between BMI and insulin sensitivity. *Journal of Endocrinological Investigation*, 25(6), pp.520-525.
- Huang, P., Fang, R., Li, B. and Chen, S., 2016. Exercise-Related Changes of Networks in Aging and Mild Cognitive Impairment Brain. *Frontiers in Aging Neuroscience*, 8.
- Kuo, Y., Song, T., Bernard, J. and Liao, Y., 2017. Short-term expiratory muscle strength training attenuates sleep apnea and improves sleep quality in patients with obstructive sleep apnea. *Respiratory Physiology & Neurobiology*, 243, pp.86-91.
- O'Connor, P., Herring, M. and Caravalho, A., 2010. Mental Health Benefits of Strength Training in Adults. *American Journal of Lifestyle Medicine*, 4(5), pp.377-396.
- Ribeiro, B., Forte, P., Vinhas, R., Marinho, D., Faíl, L., Pereira, A., Vieira, F. and Neiva, H., 2022. The Benefits of Resistance Training in Obese Adolescents: A Systematic Review and Meta-analysis. *Sports Medicine - Open*, 8(1).
- Richards, K., Lambert, C., Beck, C., Bliwise, D., Evans, W., Kalra, G., Kleban, M., Lorenz, R., Rose, K., Gooneratne, N. and Sullivan, D., 2011. Strength Training, Walking, and Social

    Activity Improve Sleep in Nursing Home and Assisted Living Residents: Randomized Controlled Trial. *Journal of the American Geriatrics Society*, 59(2), pp.214-223.

GET YOUR FREE BONUS NOW!

20 MINUTES HOME TRAINING

Printed in Great Britain
by Amazon